Kerry Jones

Parental Perspectives on Grief and Loss Following Perinatal Death

D1807183

Kerry Jones

Parental Perspectives on Grief and Loss Following Perinatal Death

LAP LAMBERT Academic Publishing

Impressum / Imprint

Bibliografische Information der Deutschen Nationalbibliothek: Die Deutsche Nationalbibliothek verzeichnet diese Publikation in der Deutschen Nationalbibliografie; detaillierte bibliografische Daten sind im Internet über http://dnb.d-nb.de abrufbar.

Alle in diesem Buch genannten Marken und Produktnamen unterliegen warenzeichen-, marken- oder patentrechtlichem Schutz bzw. sind Warenzeichen oder eingetragene Warenzeichen der jeweiligen Inhaber. Die Wiedergabe von Marken, Produktnamen, Gebrauchsnamen, Handelsnamen, Warenbezeichnungen u.s.w. in diesem Werk berechtigt auch ohne besondere Kennzeichnung nicht zu der Annahme, dass solche Namen im Sinne der Warenzeichen- und Markenschutzgesetzgebung als frei zu betrachten wären und daher von jedermann benutzt werden dürften.

Bibliographic information published by the Deutsche Nationalbibliothek: The Deutsche Nationalbibliothek lists this publication in the Deutsche Nationalbibliografie; detailed bibliographic data are available in the Internet at http://dnb.d-nb.de.

Any brand names and product names mentioned in this book are subject to trademark, brand or patent protection and are trademarks or registered trademarks of their respective holders. The use of brand names, product names, common names, trade names, product descriptions etc. even without a particular marking in this works is in no way to be construed to mean that such names may be regarded as unrestricted in respect of trademark and brand protection legislation and could thus be used by anyone.

Coverbild / Cover image: www.ingimage.com

Verlag / Publisher:
LAP LAMBERT Academic Publishing
ist ein Imprint der / is a trademark of
AV Akademikerverlag GmbH & Co. KG
Heinrich-Böcking-Str. 6-8, 66121 Saarbrücken, Deutschland / Germany
Email: info@lap-publishing.com

Herstellung: siehe letzte Seite /
Printed at: see last page
ISBN: 978-3-659-32271-6

Zugl. / Approved by: University of Bristol, Bristol, UK, 2010

Dedication

This research is dedicated to twenty-seven parents who so generously told their stories and to the memory of their children. This body of work would not have been possible without such personal experience so I dedicate it also to the memory of my daughter, *Bron*.

Acknowledgements

I wholeheartedly express my thanks to the men and women who so selflessly gave their time to tell their story and to the group facilitators who provided contact with parents. I would like to acknowledge my husband Colin Pike, my family and all my children. This research concerning the bereavement experiences of twenty-seven parents was funded by the University of Bristol scholarship and also received funding assistance from the British Sociological Association Phil Strong Memorial Prize, and the University of Bristol, Robert Skills PhD award.

She pass'd away like morning dew
Before the sun was high;
So brief her time, she scarcely knew
The meaning of a sigh.

As round the rose is soft perfume
Sweet love around her floated;
Admired she grew – while mortal doom
Crept on, unfear'd unnoticed.

(Hartley Coleridge, 'Early Death', in Quiller – Couch, 1919:751)

Doctoral Thesis Submitted to the University of Bristol, UK

Table of Contents

List of Tables

Introduction

"*And can it be in a world so full and busy, the loss of one weak creature makes a void in any heart so wide and deep that nothing but the width and depth of vast eternity can fill it up.*" (Charles Dickens, *Dombey and Son*, 1848/1995:221)

"*Give sorrow words: the grief that does not speak whispers the o'er-fraught heart and bids it break.*" (William Shakespeare, Macbeth, 1606/2005, Act IV, Scene 3:75)

Seventeen babies a day die in the UK, yet existing research suggests that stillbirth and neonatal loss remains a marginal topic (Stillbirth and Neonatal Death Society, SANDS 2009). There is a need therefore as well as scope to explore how men and women experience the stillbirth or neonatal death of their child. While the professional literature discusses such deaths, it is unclear from where these perspectives are derived, professionals or parents.

This study will therefore seek to develop a greater understanding for professionals who work with bereaved parents, adding to existing research about bereavement and the multidisciplinary orientations to understanding death and grief in contemporary western societies. Though this has particular relevance to an academic audience, it would serve further to support bereaved parents as they attempt to derive meaning from reading other men's and women's bereavement experiences.

The empirical research presented within this thesis comes from twenty-seven interviews with men and women (six men and twenty-one women).

I introduced this thesis with extracts from the works of Dickens and Shakespeare since I came to this research from my experiences as a bereaved mother. Following the neonatal death of my daughter after what was an otherwise normal, full term, pregnancy, my experience did not fit within the 'norms' of grief theory and models.

Indeed, at that moment there was very little I knew of myself or the world. Grief impacted upon every aspect of my life and ability to function, socially, relationally and as an academic researcher. I felt stuck, abnormal and unable to 'move on.' There was no reference point by which to make sense of this new world I now occupied. Any sense of normality could only be found within the confines of another group of parents who I felt knew something of this vast empty space that I occupied, and who would allow me to memorialise my precious very longed for child. Assimilating the past into the unity of my present life has been learnt slowly. I have learnt that not everything is irretrievably lost but everything is irrevocably stored and so my bond with my child continues. Though this is represented in my creative writings, journal work and in many other ways it allows me to remain connected to her and nourished in my life without her.

These bereavement experiences were for some time inextricably linked to contemporary UK health care systems. I became intrigued by these encounters both as a former researcher of dementia and as a bereaved parent. This led me to think in new ways about dialogic exchanges between professionals and patients and about the corporeal structure in which they are embedded. This enabled me to develop this thesis which explores men and women's experiences of grief and loss following stillbirth and neonatal death.

In my wider discussions with the bereaved parent community I noted that notions of grief in the bereavement literature both frustrated and aggrieved them. In developing a framework for this research, I identified the extent to which both these experiences of grief and loss were marginal topics, particularly in relation to men, where they were much less written about.

Further, the wider ramifications of this form of loss on other family members (siblings and grandparents) were at best a secondary issue in much of the literature.

Yet my discussion with men and women showed that the effects of the deaths on these relationships had implications for the well-being of bereaved parents following loss. I was unable to find a body of research which adequately addressed these important and mediating issues.

I have considered multidisciplinary orientations to understanding grief and loss and conclude that though they have relevance they are inadequate in considering the varying experiences of men and women following loss.
 contend that this owes to the sequestration of the experience more generally and to social considerations of existential issues. Chapters 1-3 of this thesis, fully explores these bodies of research, to which I now turn to discuss their relative contribution to understanding death, grief and mourning.

Multidisciplinary Approaches to Understanding Death, Grief and Loss
From this starting point it is important to distinguish my reference to grief and mourning. Following Seale (1998:198), grief can be said to describe feelings and the feeling actions of the bereaved while mourning concerns the behaviour socially prescribed in a culture as appropriate for those who are bereaved. In Chapter 1, focus is given to the body of multidisciplinary orientations which attempt to provide an understanding of death, grief and mourning. I explore these approaches within sociological discussions concerning the contradictory presence and absence of death debate in society. Consideration is given to the idea that death is a socially denied phenomenon, sequestered by medicine, yet exposed in all its rawness by the media.

The sociologist Tony Walter's (1996) social and historical understanding of death ritual and mourning is both explored and criticised. His typology attempts to define typical deaths and ways of mourning in the 'traditional', the 'modern' and more recent 'postmodern' age. I argue that the problem with this understanding is that it aligns with the ruminations of Ariès

8

(1974, 1993) and Gorer (1965) who postulate a return to 'traditional' *deathways.*

A return to past rituals is advocated by these authors since they argue that the late modern concern with grief is isolating and meaningless. Though in part I concur, a return to the past I argue requires homogeneity in society (a feature of Walter's 'traditional' *deathways*). Considered against the heterogeneity of a culturally diverse western society this holds little possibility.

Following these social historical approaches, I investigate some of the ways in which the media influences popular perceptions of death and grief in western culture and which serve to challenge the view that death is taboo and forever sequestered since it is this which has influenced sociological discussion about public responses to loss. I contend that visible death remains largely hidden from public discourse, yet, the media provide a way of presenting death which is 'othered' in that the deaths they portray happen to others and, thus, we do not have to contemplate them for ourselves.

In my discussion of the media I expose the tension in the social experience of death and its cultural expression. For this reason I argue that sociological reference to the absence or presence of death cannot be reduced to a simple dichotomy, it requires more complex considerations. I argue that these need to be viewed in light of men and women's experiences in this research.

I also consider theoretical models of grief which have been used to develop an understanding of grief from various disciplines. Until more recently, the study of grief has been the domain of psychiatry and psychology, emanating from the works of Freud (1913, 1917), Bowlby (1980), Kubler-Ross (1997) and others (Parkes, 1986, Worden, 1991, 2003).

These understandings I argue, are prescriptive and overly dominated by concerns of 'normal' and 'pathological' states that rely for their validity on a medical model. In so doing, they assume universality to experiences of grief. That this is limiting is shown by the responses of men and women in this thesis.

The literature that deals with the impact of the death of a child at all ages specifically suggests that women, in particular, experience sadness, despair, self-blame and guilt.

Studies which explore these states suggest that other mediating factors may include previous losses and levels of support. However, these studies are largely quantitative in their scope, and overlook the subtleties of the meaning of the death of a baby. This is dealt with in Chapter 2, where I fully investigate the meaning of the death of a child at different ages.

A case is made that the death of a child in childhood, adolescence or adulthood represents 'one of life's greatest tragedies' (Brown, 1989), since in the eyes of the parent, they will always be a child. I argue that these contrast to the popular view of deaths which occur in infancy, particularly following stillbirth and neonatal death, since such deaths do not receive the same social endorsements when viewed as little more than a disappointment. This is considered in light of the evolutionary psychology thesis which postulates the more you have in child years, the greater the sense of the loss. I argue that this notion is limiting and has no evidence to support it. It imposes a hierarchy of grief from which this thesis distinguishes itself.

Such losses cannot be seen as greater or less, they need to be viewed in light of their meaning which as shown in the analysis chapters (5-8), is devastating. Thus, the evolutionary psychology thesis reflects a similar

10

tendency to psychological theories, which is to marginalise social influences and how these impact on experiences of loss.

Having considered the death of children at different ages, the meaning of the death of a baby is discussed in relation to biomedical expectations of which the work of Linda Layne (2003) proffers a useful understanding. This shows that pregnancies are on the whole expected to succeed. This is informed by medicine and notions of scientific progress of which obstetric and neonatal technology can be a speciality in saving and prolonging lives. Men and women become saturated by such notions of medical progress more widely and in the media. Therefore, when medical technology fails to avert the death of a baby it is, therefore, shocking.

The impact of these losses is considered in light of marital intimacy and gendered emotional responses to loss. Voluntary organisations such as SANDS suggest that many men and women experience difficulties in their relationships within a few months of the loss of a baby. Others (Lang et al, 1996; Najman et al, 1993) suggest that these difficulties are sufficient to end some marriages. In part this is explained by differing responses to loss by bereaved parents. References to these differences postulate the notion that women are tasked with emotional expressivity (crying) while men are informed by wider discourses to remain stoic and active (organising the funerals). I challenge these assumptions on two counts since research (Riches and Dawson, 2000), points to both men and women being both emotional and engaging in activities normally associated with funerary rituals (organising the funeral service, ordering caskets).

Secondly, I argue that while these dominant discourses provide some explanation they do not consider the presence of surviving siblings within the family and some of the ways in which this mediates men and women's responses to loss. Indeed, it will be shown in chapters 5-8 that this is critical to understanding responses to loss and men and women's sense of identity.

11

From this position I consider notions of the meaning of motherhood and fatherhood and argue that they are framed by the discourses associated with them. This concerns binary categorisations of motherhood/non-motherhood and fatherhood/non-fatherhood which I argue are a crude way of defining a parent. I argue that men and women may see themselves as parents even when they have not reproduced, for example through adoption or step- parenting. What these binaries overlook are the lived experiences of men and women and the meanings they give to these experiences.

In Chapter 5, I show that men and women feel as if their identity has been taken away; they feel they have become a mother and father having contributed to the identity of the child, yet they remain childless. In this ambiguity, men and women turn to their social networks to affirm their status as bereaved parents and learn that such validation is limiting.

Giddens's (1991) ideas concerning existentialism are discussed in relation to people's responses to the bereaved more widely, in that the death of a baby represents a loss that is incomprehensible for some. I argue that this can be consequential to a parent's sense of self since their grief is disenfranchised. In incorporating these arguments, I affirm that parental and social responses to the death of a baby are multifaceted and that their expression and experience of grief is socially constructed.

Having reviewed the various literature and research concerning bereavement there were none that could adequately account for men and women's subjective experiences following loss. From my reading of Riches and Dawson's (2000) research on parental bereavement, stillbirth and neonatal death were viewed as one and the same as other child deaths. The research overlooked what is central to the experiences of bereaved men and women in this thesis.

These 'early' deaths differ in that they are not recognised by some parents' social networks as being of any significance which causes frustration and anger. Further, it is assumed more widely by these networks that having another child negates the pain of the loss of the previous child; this is a recurring theme, particularly for women, in this research. Indeed, there is limited consideration in the literature of the ways in which women may interpret these responses and of their impact. That it subsumes grief is one thing, that it is seen as a preoccupation with loss is another.

In contrast, feminist researches such as those of Layne (2003) have explored the way women give meaning to their loss through memorialisation rituals and gift giving to the deceased baby as a way to mark their significance. This informed my thinking about the way in which men and women constructed rituals on the baby's anniversary, as revealed in my research. Though this tended to happen with others in support groups, it shows another way in which men and women continue to search for meaning.

This understanding of the research permits an engagement with a parent's lived biography, without obscuring subjectivity. The potential of this approach is the recognition that men and women's embodied experiences are not separate from their overall life story, they represent a disruption, an interruption which does not separate the physical experience from the meaning. Such experiences are further explored in relation to a medical discourse concerning emotionality and death in Chapter 3.

In exploring the multidisciplinary approaches to understanding death, ritual and mourning in society (Chapter 1), and the literature about grief following the loss of a child, in Chapter 2, it is proffered that medical discourse concerning death represents a discursive framework about a form of knowledge. I argue that medicine provides a way to perceive death which has become a dominant discourse in understanding life and meaning.

One of the features of medicine in the late modern age is the role of health professionals in the management of death and dying. I consider representations of emotionality and expressivity by the profession to explain varying professional responses to loss. In so doing I explore the sociology of emotions, a sub discipline of which has attracted a number of classical debates in sociology.

I draw on the oft cited reference to Hochschild's (2003) 'emotional management' thesis. I argue that emotionality within medicine represents an element of work which is consequential to professionals and subject to the 'corporeal' feeling rules of the institutions in which they work. This sense of corporeality I argue is dependent upon a level of coherency which is limited and assists in explaining varying professional approaches to loss.

By drawing on the interactional and organismic approach of Hochschild, this consideration of the medical encounter, I contend, is a novel approach, since it considers dialogic exchanges as well as notions of power in these exchanges. It will be shown that a level of emotionality is expected in these encounters generally, yet, this notion is unsupported in the socialisation of professionals in their training.

I argue that this represents the basis of medicine more widely, the foundation of which is grounded by a rational and scientific model of emotion. These approaches are foregrounded with a discussion on the socio-political aspects of the death of a baby. Legislation, I argue, defines foetal personhood, and, thus, parental identity.

This understanding of emotions lends weight to the body of research concerning their expressivity since it is central to contemporary sociological discussion and is critical to understanding men and women's experiences.

A discussion of more recent policies by voluntary organisations is considered in relation to the work of emotion in medical encounters and to the coherency of corporeality within institutions. It will be seen by these analyses that emotions are a phenomenon which is uncontainable in any one discourse. In this respect, emotions are embodied experiences, which involve active engagement with the world and the self. The emotionally expressed body then, is the basis for self within the wider culture.

In this chapter I employ the term perinatal loss to describe the deaths of stillborn children and babies who die on the neonatal ward, as this is the language used in the literature and official statistics concerning these types of death. Synthesising these multidisciplinary approaches to understanding embodied experience has enabled me to develop an understanding of men and women's bereavement experiences.

They reflect my aims which are to:

- **Provide a more complete understanding of mothers' and fathers' narratives of grief and loss following the death of their child.**

- **Explore the ways in which parents give meaning to their experiences in light of existing discourses regarding parenthood, grief, loss, gender and medicine.**

- **Explore some of the ways in which parents continue or sever the relationship with the child who has died.**

- **Explore possible gender differences in the expression of grief following the death of a baby.**

- **Elicit insight into parents' perspectives on the care they received following the death of their child in hospital.**

15

- **Contribute to social research, health care and theoretical knowledge pertaining to parent's lived experience.**

- **Recommend appropriate policy for the care of parents following the death of their child and future research directions.**

Chapter 4 describes the way this research was carried out and the methodology employed to analyse men and women's narratives. This research is about enabling men and women to describe their experiences of grief following the death of their stillborn or neonatal child. It also explores the factors that facilitated the continuing connection to their child in their new and changed lives.

Methodological Approach

I contextualise myself in this research, in particular in the methodology section so that the reader is able to recognise my potential biases and how my knowledge of the phenomenon has informed the study. I have aimed to make sociological sense of my 'self' in the process of research in order to try and understand others' experiences. This involves recognising how I have positioned myself in relation to the research process and how this has affected the product of the research in relation to choice of design, analysis, editorship and presentation of data within this thesis.

This approach compares with traditional, academic study where researching 'others' may be viewed as an impersonal activity in which 'objective' methodological approaches are highly valued. From this 'expert' stance however, there is a distancing of the like in which sight of the researcher and their impact upon the research process and product is missing. Indeed, respondents are expected to reveal aspects (and more) of their lives and selves while we as researchers traditionally refrain from such risk taking.

This is why I value the approach of other reflexive researchers, in particular Etherington (2003), who suggests that by revealing ourselves in research we not only make deeper connections with our topic, we learn more about ourselves.

This approach to researching men and women's experiences of loss is methodologically innovative. It can be read as a reflexive study which emanates from narrative, heuristic, and auto/biographical methodologies. It is a way of researching which values emotion and men and women's subjective lived experience. To this end the voice relational method was utilised in my analyses of narratives since in reading and re-reading transcripts, the different 'voices' were uncovered. Though this seems labour intensive, I was able to remain close to the data and become immersed within it by working in a reflexive way. Thus, neither voices nor themes were obscured as in other studies of stillbirth and neonatal death.

The utility of employing the voice relational method for analysing narratives is demonstrated in Chapter 4. The method shows a way to bring out the complexities of experience that were revealed in the interviews. Here, I observed different ways in which individuals express their grief (e.g. narratives, poetry, journal entries, art work and photographs). These expressions exposed the meaning of an experience from an aspect of parents' biographies and were a way to overcome the limitations of the spoken language.

Stillbirth and neonatal death are sensitive subjects and personal to the men and women they affect. Such phenomena call for a way of researching which has at its centre the respondent as agent and as master of their own narrative.

I began the process of gaining access to respondents by contacting SANDS who provided the telephone numbers of six support group facilitators. I was able to provide written information (Appendices A to F) to these facilitators to give to men and women in their groups. Referred to more broadly as a snowball method, in that as one person was interviewed, others came forward, I obtained access to conduct twenty-seven interviews with bereaved men and women in their homes.

My original aim was to conduct thirty or more interviews. Men and women were invited to take part in this research through the information I had posted on the SANDS web site and babyloss.com, yet none were forthcoming. SANDS were approached once again to obtain the contact details of other support group facilitators in which to access more respondents but this was refused. I contend though that twenty seven interviews generated a large amount of data within which to develop an insightful understanding of men and women's experiences. To elucidate the value of these findings it is useful to summarise the basis of the four readings of the data collected from men and women.

Analysis Chapters. The Four Readings
The first reading of the data was concerned with the overall plot of men and women's narratives. These plots contextualised their experience of stillbirth and neonatal death in relation to notions of motherhood and fatherhood. This was in keeping with the aims of the research which was to describe their experiences. This approach enabled reflexivity, in that I located myself in the research. I outlined the narrative context and explored their interpretation of their embodied experience. In so doing, I retained the discourse of the respondent all along in the analysis.

In these narrative plots, there were subplots, the central part of which is the death of the child. The sub-plot represents the varying ways these stories came about. I demonstrate that they are stories told through wounded voices since they represent the emotionality of the narrator.

In this approach the words are read for as well as listened to in order to capture the silences which represent the emotionality in telling a story. Searching for truisms and competing perspectives does not fit here, it is an embodied lived experience in which I search for meaning, and how that meaning was derived. In this innovative way, men and women's voices are captured to impute an understanding of experience. The stories unfold as they are told and change as narrators bring forth the protagonists of their story.

The second reading was for the 'voice of the 'I'. Here, I consider the use of pronouns such as 'I', 'We' and 'You' which respondents employ to describe their experiences. In this chapter, I explore men and women's sense of selves and in so doing pay attention to the various voices. It is within these narratives that the utility of metaphors to describe wounding experiences is exposed.

While some men and women struggled to narrate their experiences, others provided cohesive narratives. Though the latter represent stories as part of their overall life stories, they represent a narrative part which I contend has been rehearsed. This re-telling of stories comes about in various forms, yet more often than not in support groups where it is expected these stories are shared. While it was women more than men who visited these groups, men were as able to provide narrations which came from lengthy interviews (three hours). These narratives also exposed the subtle contradictions in telling a story and represented the tension in men and women's lives. What these narratives demonstrate is that the sample of men and women interviewed in my research were distinctive in consisting of more reflexive parents who have sought support.

In the subsequent Chapter (7) concerning reading for relationships, I explore men and women's encounters with others (spouse, surviving children, relatives, colleagues and health professionals). This demonstrates that men and women's present confusion stems from their knowledge of relationships through experience and their sense of ambivalence as a parent/non-parent.

The fourth and final reading (Chapter 8) explores the wider cultural contexts and social structures within which men and women experienced their loss. Here, I explore the broader discourse that mediated men and women's experiences concerning stillbirth and neonatal death. Several accounts suggest that men and women were subjected to these dominant discourses, particularly those concerning continuing bonds.

As part of a reflexive approach to research the meaning given to these losses are made explicit by paying attention to the way within which experiences are narrated. This narrative inquiry focuses upon the language employed by men and women in relation to dominant discourses (psychological notions of grief), and the rejection and acceptance of such discourses, relationship with others (partners and relatives) and the self, coping mechanisms, bereavement support and cultural and social structures, such as employment, religion and belief system.

CHAPTER 1. Concepts of Death, Ritual and Mourning

> *"Loss of a loved person is one of the most intensely painful experiences any human being can suffer and not only is it painful to experience but it is also painful to witness, if only because we are so impotent to help. To the bereaved nothing but the return of the lost person can bring true comfort; should what we provide fall short of that it is felt almost as an insult. That, perhaps, explains a bias that runs through much of the older literature on how human beings respond to loss. Whether an author is discussing the effects of loss on an adult or a child, there is a tendency to underestimate how intensely distressing and disabling loss usually is and for how long the distress, and often the disablement, commonly lasts. Conversely, there is a tendency to suppose that a normal healthy person can and should get over bereavement not only fairly rapidly but also completely."* (Bowlby, 1980:7-8)

Introduction

A sociological understanding of death, ritual and mourning in relation to society has been influenced by several disciplines including social history, anthropology, psychology and medicine. More recently, representations of death and dying in the modern age have been portrayed by the media and in the personal grief narratives of the bereaved. This has served to challenge the debate over the absence or presence of death in public discourse which has dominated death studies for some time (Hanusch, 2008:301).

In this chapter I explore some of the ways in which western societies approach death, dying and bereavement. I consider the multidisciplinary approaches about ways of thinking about death and bereavement. In particular, consideration is given to the notion that death is denied by society, yet exposed by the media and sequestered by medicine. Attention is given to medical and psychological approaches to understanding grief, since I argue this has influenced a modern way of thinking about grief which is inadequate and contradictory to the experiences of the bereaved in the modern age.

I begin by placing these perspectives in the context of social history and in different societies since this has been central to the discussion on mortality and social responses to death.

Thus, I explore and critique Walter's (1996:195) typology of death in traditional, modern and post modern society. It will be argued that the problem with this approach is that it assumes that Western societies are essentially homogenous and share a common response to death despite the contemporary reality of a socially and culturally diverse society.

Following Walter, I explore the media as a means of influencing popular perceptions and attitudes to death and grief and some of the ways they have served to challenge the notion that death is taboo, and removed from public discourse since it is this which more recently has influenced discussions about public responses to death and dying. I argue that despite the media, visible death is still largely hidden from public discourse, yet the media provide ways of portraying death which has become 'othered', in that they are deaths which we do not expect for ourselves and, thus, do not have to contemplate. It will be shown that this reveals the tension inherent in the social experience of death and its cultural expression. For this reason, I conclude by stating that the 'absence or presence of death debate' cannot be reduced to a simple dichotomy, rather it needs to be considered in a much more complex light.

This informs later discussions regarding parental bereavement (Chapter 2). One way to deconstruct the dominant notions of bereavement is by exploring parents' own narrative accounts of grief and loss. Such experiences are explored throughout Chapter 7 and a wider discussion of the merits of employing this approach is provided in the methodology section in Chapter 4.

Sociological Approaches to Understanding Death, Grief and Mourning

A claim that death had become a hidden and forbidden phenomenon in Western societies was made by the influential French historian Ariès (1974, 1993) who argued that ours is a death denying society. For sociologists such as Gorer (1965), the extent of this absence of death from public discourse was such that it represented a form of pornography, an unmentionable and invisible part of life that had become taboo. In more recent times, research has suggested that death has returned to public discourse (Littlewood, 1992; Walter, 1994, 1999). This is based upon the premise that very public deaths such as those of key social figures and individuals (e.g. the late Princess Diana and soldiers killed fighting in Iraq and Afghanistan) are widely portrayed to mass audiences in western societies. Yet, even these authors concur that these deaths are extraordinary in that unlike most deaths which happen to citizens on a daily basis at home or in hospital, they have occurred in the public domain. This serves to contradict the idea that death has become taboo, sequestered and forever unmentioned. Of note is the lack of consideration about some of the ways in which bereaved individuals make sense of the death of a loved one and find meaning for their loss.

An understanding of death and grief within sociology raises questions about the way in which death has been constructed in relation to Western discourse. Social history has been employed in these discussions about death and ritual practices by French historians such as Ariès (1974), as well as contributions by anthropologists (Bauman, 1992) and later professionals and counsellors involved in death management within contemporary societies. Social historians, for example, have described the complexity and the centrality of funerary practices during the nineteenth century (Ariès 1974, 1981; Gorer, 1965), while health professionals have subsequently interpreted these *deathways* as being of therapeutic value in contemporary society (Ariès, 1993; Howarth, 2008).

Much of the criticism about contemporary western approaches to death stems from social history, in that traditional societies of the past are perceived as having responded to death and the needs of the bereaved through whole communities engaging in rituals which had therapeutic value for survivors. As a consequence of modernity, traditions have been relinquished and medicine embraced as progress. Thus, the central point of this debate is that the modern experience of death has become meaningless, isolating, medicalised and privatised. It therefore follows that a more recent rejection of medical and scientific rationale signifies a change in responses to death in contemporary society and a quest for finding more humane ways to comprehend loss (Howarth, 2008).

To explore some of the ways sociologists perceive the absence or presence of death in relation to society, Walter (1996:34) argues that it is necessary to consider changes in responses to death in the context of different societies. Walter compares and contrasts three different types of death in relation to what he defined as traditional, modern and postmodern society as a way of explaining how this has fed into the dominant discourses about death available to contemporary society.

Death in traditional society

A traditional society for Walter is characterised by a high death rate and high infant mortality rate. His model essentially represents an agrarian society bound by a religious culture which had authority in ritual and language about death. Walter suggests that death in this phase was mainly caused by infectious disease such as the plague which affected entire communities and eradicated its victims with speed and unpredictability. Walter suggests that death in the traditional phase is typified by community. By this he means that people lived in the same neighbourhood for all of their lives and thus, each death was publicly mourned. Yet it is argued that this may not have been viable at a time of important historical and social change in nineteenth century England. The industrial revolution in England bore witness to the mass movement of people from community villages to towns and cities to work in factories and mills.

Though infectious disease was virulent in cities it varied across the social landscape and between the middle and working classes. For example, in England in 1842 the average age of life for labourers in the city was seventeen years of age compared to professionals whose life expectancy approximated thirty eight years of age (Archer, 1999). These changes showed that whole families and communities were separated as people sought to find work, which meant that the ability to care for the sick, dying and dead was diminishing (Kellehear, 2007). This would suggest that another phase was emerging which typified the way people experienced death and responded to loss.

Modern deathways

In contrast to Walter's notion of the experience of death and cultural expression in his traditional society, in the second period, modern society he perceives a shift in authority from religion to medical experts which is associated with improved nutrition, clean water and curative medicine. Babies are expected to thrive into adulthood, while those who die, do so from deaths which linger (cancer, heart disease). Death is not so much in people's lives since its management has extended to the funeral industry and away from public view.

In Walter's modern society, there is an emphasis upon reconstructing individual identity following loss by engaging in a 'grief process' that has been defined and prescribed by an 'expert'. Unlike the idea of the 'traditional' phase of authority on how to mourn, meaning is not given by the church and prayer or other public bodies, as a means of coping but by the 'experts' that is the health professionals and the therapists.

This is an interesting concept which I explore in Chapter 2 and discuss in Chapter 7 following parents' accounts of loss which reject such knowledge. This is in keeping with a more post modern way of thinking about grief in that it provides ways by which the bereaved can identify and choose what suits their needs.

Postmodern death and dying

Walter's notion of the experience of death in a postmodern society represents the later part of the twentieth century and is characterised by a rationalised form of death where the cause is known, the outcome is specific and information about it is shared. This represents a shift in attitudes to death for Walter, since the expression of grief is now influenced by advanced technology which serves to link people with similar interests. For example, mutual self-help groups and websites depicting narratives on loss provide a forum for bereaved people to share their grief and act as a legitimate source by which they can reconstruct their damaged identity. Walter posits that this more contemporary phase is about the individual mourner who is the ultimate authority on their own experience and of finding ways to express their sorrow.

Thus, Walter's perspective suggests that religion forms the basis to provide meaning and understanding in traditional society, whereas in modern societies medical science has replaced religion as an authority on understanding life. In postmodern societies, both religion and medicine have been usurped by the individual as the authority on the self with an emphasis on therapy. For Walter, this represents a significant shift in the social and cultural expression of grief since it is publicly shared. Yet it is argued that what has changed is with *whom* that grief is shared and the *location* of its expression. The neighbour or community helper who once may have helped to prepare the corpse for burial may not be the shoulder to cry on when the burden of grief is too much to bear.

Rather, it could be argued that it is the stranger in the guise of a funeral director who attends to the body of a person that is sorely missed, and it is the mourner who might seek out an understanding of the situation from others with similar bereavement experiences (e.g. bereavement narratives, World Wide Web forums).

Walter's perspective is limited to identifying some (not all) approaches rather than dominant attitudes towards death in traditional, modern or post modern societies. Walter's ideas about death and changes in responses to loss utilise broad categories and as a consequence are unable to reveal the complexity within each society itself. Moreover, societies cannot be placed so precisely into distinct historical or anthropological phases since practices or types of death do not fit neatly into any of the categories. For example, Walter's concept of a traditional society incorporates all societies which have yet to industrialise. This groups contemporary agrarian societies with European medieval communities and those of the Ancient Egyptians by suggesting that pastoral people were subject to death by infectious disease.

As Kellehear (2007:79) notes, while waves of epidemics visited such societies, they were often accompanied by large scale scapegoating and mortal recriminations. Without biological explanations, burnings, drowning, torture and imprisonment of women (witch hunts), and minority groups (Jews), travelling strangers and homosexuals were commonplace. Moreover, in China, Egypt, Africa and Mesoamerica human sacrificial offerings was a major cause of death (Kellehear, 2007). This suggests that for some pastoral people, epidemic misery preceded death, whereas for others it was the life threatening human sacrifices which had to be avoided.

In more modern societies, medicine may be at the forefront of understanding illness and death, yet religious beliefs continue for many as a source of comfort and as a way of understanding mortality. In contemporary western societies the dominance of medicine has not disappeared. Indeed, people still have a faith in medicine in the hope that it may cure all ills. Moreover, there is significant social and cultural diversity such that there are multitudes of ways by which the bereaved impute meaning to their loss. For example, recently the media televised a High Court decision to grant a UK citizen the right to have her body burnt on an open pyre following death.

For others, (Byrne, 2008; Chitty, 2009) comfort and meaning is sourced from psychic phenomena, a concept I explore in Chapter 8 in relation to continuing bonds with the deceased.

Yet despite reference in the literature as to the therapeutic value of traditional ways of mourning, a contemporary and therefore postmodern way of managing death and grieving does not imply a return to tradition. Rather, it is a postmodern individual who is the authority on the self and chooses what suits them best. The key point to make here is that Walter views religion, medicine and psychology as dominant discourses which reflect the power of different social groups. Yet it is argued there are more recent discourses which while less visible are of equal importance. The voices of women, men and the working classes in relation to mortality reflect this diversity (see Keaggy, 2002, Don, 2005, Finkenbeiner, 1996 respectively).

Aside from Walter, other explanations for the changes in death in relation to society suggest that with declining death rates in the twentieth century, people felt less of a need to ritualise (Howarth, 2008). While this decline does not account for World War I (1914-18) and later World War II (1939-1945), it suggests that in the ensuing decades people kept their grief to themselves. That was until the 1960s when a culture of freedom of self-expression developed which could be applied not only to socio-political issues but also to attitudes to death and dying.

This shift in thinking about mortality found its way into new approaches in sociological research which emphasised individual agency and meaning and experiences. For example, sociologists such as Glaser and Strauss (1967) in the United States, concerned with the presumed silence surrounding death and medicalised forms of dying, generated a new discourse to free dying people from the taboo by which they had become bound. For Glaser and Strauss and later Illich (1977), the problems of dying in modern societies emanate from institutions which emphasise scientific medical solutions as a cure at the expense of palliative care.

These ideas compare with Gorer's and Ariès' arguments cited earlier in this chapter that the problems of dying and social responses to the event emanate from a loss of traditions. Others such as Becker (1973) argue that societies are death denying in response to fears about mortality.

The concept of death denying societies is interesting since it assumes that a change in traditional ritual *deathways* represents a denial of death in society. Yet the concept of death denied is important to the death debate in sociological discussions about mortality, since it assumes that knowledge of death is obtained by the extent to which society is exposed to it. Of note is the extent to which the media provide representations and images of death in newspapers, and on television. Upon this basis, it is critical to consider the notion that the media in some way shape public perceptions and attitudes towards death and grief by providing a profile and very strong visual images about death and dying. Some forms of death such as those of key public figures and contemporary soldiers are publicised and ritualised (i.e. soldiers funeral procession in Wotton Bassett, Wiltshire), while other types of death such as neonatal death are silenced and denied.

Death, Grief and the Media

Sociological writers such as Jon Davies (1996) argue that the media fundamentally shape popular attitudes and beliefs and act as a determining cultural constraint due to the images they portray which are absorbed by audiences. For Howarth (2008:102), the media are resources that may be used in everyday narratives of culture and self-identity. The media present cultural scripts that are selectively adapted to the social context of the individual. In this respect, the media is the marker of popular cultures and social mores about death and dying. For Hockey (1997), they represent the other and not the self, since it is the other which is contemplated and which provides a safe way of thinking about death and its impact (Hockey, 1997). Indeed, death is visualised in terms of blood, war and more recently earthquakes (Haiti, January, 2010), all which serve to distance death from our own lives in the west.

Arguably, it is a news discourse which presents a way of thinking about death in a bid for sensationalism and audience and which serves to highlight, for many people in western society, a potentially threatening yet hidden aspect to life.

Part of the contradiction about the public and private death dichotomy in the media's portrayal of death, is that it bears very little resemblance to the reality of death and dying in contemporary society. For example, Gorer, writing in 1955, argues that the media have become obsessed with the portrayal of violent death since it has replaced sex as a source of entertainment. Gorer (1955) bases his arguments on the premise that since sexual pornography was produced in the Victorian era, and death subsequently silenced in the twentieth century, this led to the 'pornography of death' such that the media were compelled to portray sensationalist images of death, in particular in film. This can be seen with the proliferation of movies in the 1950s in which cowboys and Indians were slaughtered. Later, gangster movies such as the iconic 'The Godfather' portrayed gruesome vengeful deaths.

The popularity of murder mysteries (Poirot, Agatha Christie), and US soaps about the funeral industry (Six Feet Under) and more recently, vampire movies portray death which to a large extent do not happen to 'us', but to others in an alien world. Thus, while it may be uncomfortable to observe, it is not the type of death that the audience expects for themselves, such that death has become 'othered', that is, it happens to others and is not something which we need contemplate for ourselves (Howarth, 2008).

Other genres of death narrative have followed war which emphasised its effects as opposed to grief per se and of public opposition to conflict (Vietnam 1960s, 1970s). Elsewhere, the media and entertainment industry considered issues about life after death and continuing bonds with the deceased such as in the British made film, 'Truly Madly Deeply'.

Films such as this suggest that the bond between the dead and the living continue, albeit beyond the external world. Death, in some respects, has been imbued with a gentle regard in which the dead come back to guide and guard the living. Following an ethical stance more recently, the media have brought to our attention moral questions about death such as euthanasia and terminal illness through interviews with individuals and their families. Indeed, death is a constant feature in the everyday life of the viewer, the reader and listener. For example, the daily sad toll of reporting soldiers' lives lost fighting in Afghanistan and the case of the abusive death of baby Peter in the UK invoked sadness and horror among audiences. Arguably, such representations cannot be defined as representing a normal death or usual social practice.

Sociologists such as Jon Davies, (1996) and later Glennys Howarth (2008) note that there has been an increase in images of death in the media (television, newspaper, cinema) at a time when direct contact with the deceased has decreased. Even when such images are less obvious (death notices and obituaries) the media provide a cultural script which the individual selectively adopts and adapts into the social context of their world (Howarth, 2008:113). This is significant in the context of understanding social responses to death which produces specific forms of consciousness and knowledge that affect our experience and interpretation of the world.

The proliferation of death in the media challenges the notion that death has all but disappeared from public discourse and despite the popular cinematic fervor for violent endings, some portrayals of death and dying resonate with everyday experiences of death in contemporary western societies for example terminal illness. Despite the best efforts of the media to bring death into the living rooms of millions of Britons, there is a continuing tension between the experience of death and the expression of loss such that the cultural script for mourning is limited and that the current revival of interest in death receives attention from academics interested in this field.

31

What remain are very strong images of death which leave in their wake confusion and contradiction about how to respond to the bereaved. This has shown that death is multifaceted and complex and cannot be simplified into neat distinctions about what constitutes the presence or absence of death in society or how individuals respond in varying ways to grief. Given these discussions, considerations of the psychological and medical perspectives about death and bereavement which have underpinned counselling practices are critical to furthering an understanding of modern ideas about grief in western society and how it is experienced. This is important in the context of the idea considered earlier in this chapter, that it is the self who is the expert on grief in post modern societies, a perception which is discussed in relation to the parents' accounts of loss in chapters 5-8.

Psychological Approaches to Grief

"For too long a time-for half a century in fact- psychiatry tried to interpret the human mind merely as a mechanism, and consequently the therapy of mental disease a technique. I believe this dream has been dreamt. What now begins to loom on the horizon are not the sketches of a psychologized medicine but rather those of a humanized psychiatry." **(Frankl, 2006:133)**

Much of the literature which has informed grief theory and research approaches is founded upon medical and psychoanalytical models, deriving from the works of Freud (1913), *Mourning and Melancholia,* his early lectures on psychoanalysis (1917) and Bowlby's (1980), *Attachment Theory.* Other authors (Kubler-Ross,1997; Parkes, 1986, and Worden, 1991) have added to this body of knowledge to attest that the purpose of grief for the individual is a matter of working through a barrage of emotions including, anger, depression, guilt, sadness and a whole host of other feelings which the bereaved may experience. This view of grief has been widely accepted in the twentieth century, and holds that successful resolution to grief comes about by disengaging from the deceased, and 'moving on' and 'letting go' of the past (Klass,1996:4).

32

In this view, a continuation of the bond with the person who has died is symptomatic of experiencing psychological problems. While this model of grief is a twentieth century phenomenon, much of the clinical and prescriptive view of grief work has been criticised (Armstrong, 1994; De Swaan, 1990; Foucault, 1975, 1984; Rose, 1994). These models continued to be employed despite contrary evidence as to their therapeutic value and this has led in recent years to the concept of finding ways to continue the bond with the deceased.

In writing about bereavement, several writers (Stroebe, 1992; Stroebe et al, 1996:32; Marwitt and Klass, 1996:297) argue that dominant Western considerations of grief have influenced the clinical strategies employed in modern practices. One of the key characteristics of this cultural modernism is an emphasis upon reason and a faith in progress, such that the approach to life is one of efficiency and rationality (Gergen, 1994). Upon this basis, psychology has come to view the person as a machine of functionality which, when applied to grief, means that the sufferer is required to recover from intense emotions and return to their pre bereaved and 'normal' state swiftly. Grief then is a debilitating state to be overcome since it interferes with life and has to be worked through a number of tasks to achieve normality. The breaking of ties and bonds to the deceased is viewed as constituting a product of successful resolution to grief.

It is suggested that this modern way of thinking about grief emanated from Freud's (1913/57) book *Mourning and melancholia*. In his later lectures, in 1917 he argues that the bereaved person's libidinal energy remains attached to the thoughts and memories of the deceased, the *cathexis* (attachment) *to the lost object* (the deceased) needs to be withdrawn in order for the person to replenish their energy: "*Each single one of the memories and situations of expectancy which demonstrate the libido's attachment to the lost object is met by the verdict of reality that the object no longer exists.*" (1973: 255) The ties are severed by a process of detachment which Freud defined as *hypercathexis*.

33

Freud viewed the psychological function of grief work as a way of achieving freedom from an attachment to the deceased through gradual detachment and by reviewing the past memories of the deceased. The process ends when the energy devoted to the lost object (deceased) is withdrawn and transferred to new attachments. Those who fail to *hypercathect* remain emotionally stunted (Freud, 1973:245).

Freud's ideas have been influential on modern ways of thinking about grief, and he remains one of the key contributors to psychoanalytical approaches to loss in Western society (McCleod, 2008).

Freud's theoretical positioning is of interest since Freud was unable to form new attachments following significant deaths in his own life. Freud's difficulty with mourning the death of his daughter Sophie at the age of twenty seven, and later, her son at the age of four, revealed the real dilemma created by a modern world view (Silverman and Klass, 1996). This is evident in the following extracts from a letter written by Freud: *"The sweet habit of existence will see to it that things go on as before. Quite deep down I can trace the feeling of a deep narcissistic hurt that is not to be healed. My wife and Annerl are terribly shaken in a more human way."* (Freud, 1929, quoted in Jones, 1957:20)

While Freud's words clearly imply emotional pain, he does not yield to expressing this distress and instead 'copes' as he writes in another letter, by repressing his emotions: " *It is such a paralyzing event, which can stir no afterthoughts when one is not a believer and so is spared all conflicts that go with that. Blunt necessity, mute submission."* (Freud, 1929, quoted in Jones, 1957:19) Freud's submissive state continued, as did the continuing experience of the pain of loss and the inability of severing ties with his deceased loved ones.

In a letter to a friend, Ludwig Binswanger, following the news that his friend's own son had died, Freud wrote: *"Although we know that after such a loss the acute state of mourning will subside, we also know we shall remain inconsolable and will never find a substitute. No matter what may fill the gap, even if it be filled completely, it nevertheless remains something else. And actually this is how it should be. It is the only way of perpetuating that love which we do not want to relinquish."* (Freud, 1929, quoted in Jones, 1957: 92)

Evidently, Freud recognised that grief could and did last a lifetime, such that there was no end to grief work which culminated in the detachment with the past and the cutting of ties with the deceased in order to form new attachments. On the contrary, he experienced the fact of the deaths in his life with a depression deeply felt and which was publicly expressed with stoicism. Yet his writings about his own experiences with grief and later works with metapsychology were not integrated into subsequent generations of theory and research. It is Freud's early writings which informed and dominated post-Freudian paradigms of grieving. Such theories continued with the trajectory of severing the bond with the deceased, thereby forming new attachments.

Prior to John Bowlby, the late British psychiatrist, there were few who challenged Freud's notion of man's formulation of attachments as emanating from unconscious desires. Bowlby's attachment theory follows from his observations which began in 1956 of infants and children in hospitals who had become separated from their mothers as a result of illness. The premise for Bowlby's (1980) attachment thesis and ideas about separation anxiety (1998) stems from the assumption that during healthy development (of the infant and child), attachment behaviour by the child leads to the development of affectional bonds, initially between child and parent (Bowlby, 1980).

Loss of the attachment figure (parent) represents significant anxiety since it places us into the realms of separation anxiety felt as children (Bowlby,1998:85). This is in part relieved by the sense that the person will be there to respond when needed (they return) and it is this sense that acts to continue the bond and relationship for the child with their adult. Death however is deemed to nullify the possibility of the reunion between a child and its parent. Therefore, loss means having to undertake a psychological transition in which we are forced to change our view of the self and our view of the world.

While the continuation and discontinuation of bonds is much discussed in the bereavement literature (Silverman and Klass, 1996; Walter, 1996), attachment theory presupposes that the attachment behavioural system is an organized set of biologically based behaviours that is activated at times of threat, leading the individual to re-establish proximity to an attachment figure (Bowlby 1998:85).

For Bowlby then, the bereaved do not fully realise the permanence of the death of a loved one; rather the bereaved view the deceased as a person who is missing (the person has only moved into the next room - 'not lost but gone before'. It is only at the "protest phase" that a separation reaction is marked by distress with an attempt to re-establish close ties with the deceased, in this instance the attachment figure.

Such a reaction as 'separation distress' implies that in the early stages following death the permanence of loss is not fully realised or indeed understood (Bowlby, 1980). With the distress of separation, it is assumed that there is an overwhelming urge by the bereaved to search for the person who has died. For example this may mean that the bereaved person keeps all possessions of the person who has died as a way of establishing close proximity with the deceased.

When the phase of attempting to re-establish proximity with the deceased fails (they are not coming back), Bowlby (1980) posits that the next phase is the 'despair stage' where depression and withdrawal from society is symptomatic of accepting the finality of the loss. Arguably, attachment continues even with successful grief adaptation and therefore with the acceptance of the permanence of the death, which can be understood in Bowlby's (1980) final reorganisation phase.

Here, the internalizing of the deceased occurs to create meaning, identity, and a connection with the past (Marwitt and Klass, 1996; Attig, 2001; Neimeyer, 1999). This is therefore about having a mental representation of the deceased as a source of comfort rather than seeking the physical representation of the person who has died (Walter,1996).

While Bowlby's theory is widely applied by psychoanalysts in their work with the bereaved, his assumptions regarding bereavement have been criticised (Wortman and Silver 1989). He views attachment theory as being applicable to all forms of separation be it adult to adult relationships or that between a mother and child. By this he means there is little difference in terms of impact for example, between a person who has lost their spouse to that of a mother whose child has died (Bowlby, 1980:122).

In recognizing the popularity of Freud's idea, Kubler-Ross (1997) applied the resolution of grief thesis in her work with the dying. First published in 1969, her ideas would prove influential in the training curriculum of counsellors' supporting the bereaved. These perspectives can be viewed in the context of the medicalisation of death and contribute to an understanding of grief as a process to be experienced in a linear format.

Medicalisation of Death and Grief

"Mourning, a socially prescribed set of public behaviours, has been replaced by something called 'the grief process' – a prescribed set of inner feelings. Advice to bereaved people now stems not from the rules of social etiquette but from expert knowledge about the work that must be done by the individual psyche." **(Walter, 1994: 34)**

Several authors (Atkinson, 1995; Rose, 1994; Walter, 1994) argue that medical discourse considers the patient as an object of disease, where the feeling about the experience of loss is replaced by the institutionalisation of routine. Further, the influence of psychiatrists Dr Kubler-Ross and Dr Colin Murray Parkes has fed into counselling approaches and nursing practices within medicine. They argue that the person as a patient is not only a physical object of scrutiny to be cured of ill health, but also a patient who is encouraged to talk, since the only way in which the needs of the person can be further explored is through the mind. To do this one has to be encouraged to open up, talk and be listened to by the practitioner that is, by the 'expert' (Leon, 2005).

However, the dominant medical view that the dying and bereaved would not want to talk since it would prove too painful is interestingly acknowledged in Kubler-Ross's original work of interviews with three hundred patients dying from cancer. Observing the attitudes of the medical carers, she posits that while the nurses took some persuading to enable access to talk with patients about their experiences, it was the doctors who were the least reluctant to view the patient as an individual who may want to discuss their feelings about dying. From disease to feeling, the person became seen as an experiencing vehicle and the focus of enquiry their psyche. Indeed, Kubler-Ross's research on death and dying can be analysed as an experiment in which people dying from cancer were interviewed and observed by students through a glass screen.

What may be seen as an observation in which to learn how to listen to the dying can also be viewed as a reconstruction of the traditional 'anatomy lesson' where the patient is gazed at by others. From her subsequent detailed meta stories from interviews with three hundred dying patients, Kubler-Ross (1997) concluded that there were five stages of emotional responses of those patients diagnosed with terminal cancer : -

- **Denial**: shock at the diagnosis, it can't be.
- **Anger**: Why me? Why not the person who smokes 80 a day?
- **Bargaining:** I'll go to church more often if you cure me.
- **Depression**: the realisation that there is nothing anyone can do?
- **Acceptance**: the patient awaits death silently, and with good grace with little emotional support from family or friends.

To cope with one's mortality is to express feelings about dying if death is not to be feared but finally accepted by both the patient and their carer. While Kubler-Ross (1997) does accept that not all patients will enter all five stages, the model represents a prescriptive linear format which has been transferred to the counselling literature. Indeed, it is a text that is easily absorbed for nursing and medical students as a tool to prepare them in their work in palliative care but which cannot necessarily be equated with the majority of patients' experiences (Arney and Bergen, 1984:49). Dr Colin Murray Parkes (1986:27) and later Worden (1991, 2003) followed with similar stage theories of grief. While these authors acknowledge (as with Kubler-Ross) that people are individuals and that the extent to which each stage is experienced will vary enormously, the process of grief is clearly observed and viewed as a psychological process to be worked through. Grief is presumed to be a concept that is understood and a process which can be controlled.

There is a tendency to underestimate the impact and the meaning of loss in terms of its distressing and disabling effects. The prevailing assumption is that a person should get over bereavement rapidly and completely (Bowlby, 1980:8). This suggests that despite acknowledging the family context, the approaches remain essentially individualistic and privatised, and imply an acceptance of a modern western, rational, middle class society. The autonomous ability to relate to others is viewed as evidence of well being. This fails to acknowledge a range of belief systems which accept the continuing existence of the deceased and the social behaviours in which some of these relationships continue. Moreover, people who are significant to the bereaved remain influential and important whether they are physically present or absent.

Such normative concepts of grief have been criticised, in particular by Rodger and Cowles (1991) in their review of 401 journal articles. These authors argue that the literature failed in its attempts to define grief. Other authors (Bonanno and Keltner, 1997; Wortman, and Silver, 1989) are similarly disenchanted as Rodger and Cowles (1991) by the traditional process of grief model. They argue that not only has there been a failure to clearly define grief work, but the assumed benefits of working through of emotions and 'getting over it' are not supported empirically. In fact, several research reviews suggest that there is a tendency to prescribe interventions which are at best ineffective and in some instances harmful (Neimeyer, 1999).Therapists such as Leon (2005:2), concur with the critique of the medicalisation of grief. His criticism stems from concern over the use of randomised control trials to measure effective outcomes in therapy. This he argues leads to a style of psychotherapy which subordinates the therapeutic relationship to technique. By this he means that practices have been reduced to textbook versions about how to relate to the bereaved at the expense of more humane and personal understanding of the therapeutic encounter.

The central argument so far has suggested that the way grief has come to be viewed over time is as a process to be worked through according to the terms set out by 'experts'. Why is this? Grief has evolved in the twentieth century as a medical phenomenon worthy of scrutiny and as a result, a process to be managed. It has come to be viewed as a symptom which shares characteristics with depressive illnesses, and as such is a subject worthy of study by medical science (Engel, 1961). Interestingly, the most notable authors of studies on grief have been psychiatrists (Freud, 1957; Bowlby, 80; Kubler–Ross, 1997, and Parkes, 1986) who have medically prescribed what they assume to be a healthy process of grieving. That is to appreciate the permanent separation of the deceased from the bereaved in every day life. Arguably, if it is the role of experts to prescribe to the bereaved, then it can be seen that it is also the role of medicine (according to the orthodox medicalisation critique) to subjugate its patients or 'consumers' for the benefit of society (Armstrong, 1994; De Swaan, 1990; Foucault, 1975, 1984; Rose, 1994:6-8).

In the context of the debate concerning bereavement, the social purpose of a medicalised approach to bereavement is to ensure that people's grief does not become a 'social problem'. Indeed, as the prescriptive grief work suggests, the whole aim is to produce 'docile bodies' in which people are returned to normality and as 'useful citizens' as quickly as possible by the experts who act as agents of social control in society (Foucault, 1975). Posited this way, medical power is a resource by which illness and disease is identified and then managed and understood in the context of a belief system which is shaped through social, economic and political relations. This system provides guidelines whether we are physically ailing or grieving. Therefore: *"The central strategies of disciplinary power are observation, examination, measurement and the comparison of individuals against an established norm, bringing them into a field of visibility."* (Lupton, 2000: 99)

This view reflects medicalised notions as to the purpose of grief work which is to return the bereaved back to normal mode of production, and which, it is argued, is the way the medical profession handles grief. Medicine is presumed to subjugate human agency as though the 'docile body' as observed through the clinical gaze, is unable to return or manipulate the stare of the dogmatic practitioner. Influential as medicine may be, it is assumed to exist and control citizens at all levels as though there is no escape (Lupton, 2000). While attempts may be made to obtain power through persuasion by the practitioner, it does not follow that this power will be successfully exerted. Moreover, these ideas fail to acknowledge the interpersonal aspects of the medical encounter, for example, its emotional dimensions and the existence of mutual dependencies that doctors and patients have on one another and how people respond to power strategies.

The power relationship between the medical practitioner and lay person is infinitely more complex and worthy of in-depth investigation. Consideration needs to be given to the ontology of experience and to variables such as gender, cultural and social norms, age, emotional dimensions, and individuals' accumulated embodied experiences (Lupton, 2000:104). This raises questions about the diverse responses to strategies of discipline used by the medical profession and the contradiction that exists in the way people respond to medical practitioners. Indeed, the proliferation of narrative accounts of grief written by survivors of loss in the last thirty years is in part a response to this. This may suggest that rather than being 'policed' in their grief, the bereaved are rejecting the very medical discourses which have been accused of trying to contain and control them. By writing personalised and individualistic accounts of their grief (Don, 2005; Keaggy, 2002), are not the survivors reclaiming their story, their loved ones and in the case of grief, their minds? This challenges traditional approaches which suggest that the bereaved need to withdraw emotionally from the deceased and that a failure to do so is evidence of pathological symptoms.

If re-writing one's story (as the literature suggests) is the new vogue in grief work, a consideration of these more recent approaches in particular, the concept of continuing bonds with the deceased is required.

Reconstructing Grief: Continuing Bonds

Modern theories about death and grief have emphasized a 'disenfranchisement from relationship' to the deceased such that this way of thinking is not only: - *"Disrespectful to the dead person but can also produce unnecessary misery for the living."* (Hedtke, 2002: 288) Consequently such approaches have been criticised in favour of a social model of understanding grief, since increasing evidence based research has signified that death and grief are not experiences which end with a detachment from the deceased (Hedtke, 2002; Neimeyer, 1999). In the context of bereavement the loss of a significant other does not seem able to sever that bond or lead to detachment in the survivor. Yet the bereaved may be viewed as being preoccupied with the death when they continue to find a place for the deceased in their lives (Klass, 1996:197).

This has led Hedtke and other important writers on grief such as Klass (1996) and Neimeyer (1999) to promote more humanistic ways of understanding grief through the concept of continuing bonds. They suggest that people who experience the death of a loved one, rather than detach from the deceased, actually need to continue to talk about them, especially to people who knew the individual who has died. For example, by talking with others about the deceased a story is constructed and one which can be returned to at any juncture to be reflected upon, through the survivor's lifetime. This approach implies that a healthy resolution to grief is achieved by maintaining a relationship to the deceased such that it co-exists with the ongoing interactions of the survivor's daily life, while they re evaluate their self identity (Klass, 1996:197).

While the concept of continuing bonds are a comfort and serve as a way of coping, the construction of stories about the deceased's activities (funny or otherwise) while alive is not necessarily a practice which may be shared in all bereavement situations, for example, by parents who experience the death of their child during or soon after birth.

The idea of continuing the relationship with the deceased embraces the individuality of the bereaved by acknowledging the emotional consequences for the survivor and their family. Further, the continuing bonds approach appreciates the complexities involved in adapting to loss by recognising how others (family, friends, and professionals) respond to the loss. This focus on grief work centres upon adapting the relationship to the deceased (which can last a lifetime) rather than loss and detachment. Indeed, grief is viewed in light of its complexities and in oscillating between the demands of living and forging new ways of integrating the deceased in daily life. This more humane way of thinking about grief reflects the way bereavement support groups operate more widely in the community.

Conclusion

Before turning to the impact of the death of children at all ages in Chapter 2, it is useful to reflect upon the main themes pertaining to death, ritual and mourning in society. This chapter has shown that the theoretical contribution to death and dying is complex, not least because it transcends several disciplines and sub-disciplines. Of concern to sociologists is the debate about the presence or absence of death in society which they presumed could explain social responses to loss. Both Ariès and Gorer argue that western societies are death-denying, and that the problems in facing mortality and grief emanate from a loss of rituals which were prominent in traditional societies and would have therapeutic value in contemporary society. Yet both Ariès and Gorer fail to acknowledge that modern western societies are both socially and culturally heterogeneous and are marked by plural belief systems.

Walter's understanding of the changing nature of death was categorised into types of society. I argued that Walter's perspective was limited to identifying ritual approaches rather than social attitudes towards death. The practices or ways of thinking about death do not fit neatly into distinctive types and as a consequence he is unable to reveal the complexity within society itself or the presence of alternative discourses which have been marginalized, for example the voices of women, ethnic minorities and the working classes. Further, the shifting boundary of gender, nationality and class imply that there is no homogenised way of experiencing, grieving and being supported through the death of another.

Despite new approaches to researching death and dying in the late twentieth century, sociologists such as Gorer maintained that societies continued to be death-denying. This was strongly contested by media portrayals of tragic deaths of key public figures and those which occurred through war or abusive behaviour. Where this was felt insufficient exposure, it was argued, that society could pay to view death through the film industry as a source of entertainment. This alone served to challenge the notion that death was absent in society.

The media provide a discourse of a way of thinking about death, such that it becomes 'othered', in that the deaths the audience are exposed to are those they do not have to contemplate since they do not happen to ordinary citizens. Yet more recently, television documentaries about deaths of ordinary citizens (terminal illness) challenge this 'otherness' about death since they affect many people. What remain are very strong images which are contradictory to the society and culture in which the audience lives and as a consequence, there is confusion about how best to respond to mortality and to grief.

Equally contradictory are psychological approaches to grief, in particular those emanating from the psychoanalytical works of Freud which later influenced clinical practice. This was despite Freud's own difficulty with mourning which served to challenge the notion that bonds with the deceased had to be severed. The important point here is that the psychological approach was not about analysing society, but the individual bereaved person who was prescribed a grief process. It is this way of thinking about grief work which was later rejected by some individuals and which is explored in relation to parents' experiences of grief in this thesis.

The idea that the individual in postmodern society was an authority on the self was considered in relation to medicine. This focused upon the power relationship between the medical profession and the patient, with the latter assumed to be a docile body. It was argued that this relationship was more subtle and mutually dependent, such that the bereaved could ignore the response of the professional (sensitive or insensitive) yet utilise medical technology and skill to prolong life. This suggests that other than the dominant discourses there are areas of public social experience which may explain social attitudes to death.

Collectively these approaches reveal that the social response to death is multifaceted and complex and cannot be simplified into neat distinctions about what constitutes the presence or absence of death in society or what are public/private responses to grief (professional or otherwise). Sociological perspectives on grief and loss recognise that such experiences are profoundly social. In order to understand bereavement, the notion that grief is universally experienced needs to be rejected and instead, emphasis given to the social construction of loss in the light of its cultural diversity.

In the following chapters, these ideas are explored in relation to parental grief, (associated with death of a child at any age and then stillbirth and neonatal deaths), such that experiences of loss are viewed according to gendered responses to the death of a child (Chapter 2) and in relation to the responses of health professionals (Chapter 3). It is argued that a useful way of exploring men's and women's experience of the death of their child is by analysing their narrative accounts of loss in keeping with contemporary research methods (Chapters 4-8).

What is suggested in the next chapter is that while research has concerned itself with parents' responses to loss in terms of pathological symptoms, less emphasis has been given to men's and women's every day experiences of the relationships they engage in or the discourses which they are exposed to, yet which may serve to mediate their expression of loss and, thus, their ability to reconstruct their damaged self-identity.

CHAPTER 2. Grief and Loss Following the Death of a Child

> *"There seems to be no 'good' age at which a child dies, at least not in the eyes of the bereaved mother. Her investment in the child at any age, her hopes and plans for the future, and her memories of the past all contribute to a deep sense of loss and longing 'for just a few more years.''* **(Schatz, 1986: 307)**
>
> *To lose one's parent is a natural phenomenon, to experience the death of a child is not normative and therefore viewed as "life's greatest tragedy."* **(Brown, 1989: 466)**

Introduction

In Chapter 1 it was argued that people's exposure to varying discourses of death and grief was contradictory and that while socially death was a hidden phenomenon, the media were exposing death in all its rawness to society. This contrasts with the medical and psychoanalytical discourse which served to dehumanize the experience of loss by its reference to pathological and symptomatic language for example depression, despair, anxiety and which rendered bereavement a meaningless and private endeavour. By largely rejecting this way of grieving, it was assumed that medicine was less influential on the bereaved in the later decades of the twentieth century. Yet this could not explain people's continuing faith in medical progress and their experience of disillusionment when it failed to prolong life. More recently, it was sociologically proffered that we were witnessing a revival of interest in death, yet this was contested as being confined to the interested few and not the mass public. What remains is that with the exception of sociologists (Frost, 2004; Howarth, 2008), there is limited understanding about why people varyingly accept and reject the dominant discourses of grief, or why society provides the resources for grieving, yet constrains its expression.

In this chapter I explore the meaning of the death of a child and some of the ways in which parents respond to loss, by first examining the evolutionary psychology thesis. This approach imposes a hierarchy of grief such that the death of an infant is viewed as disappointing, while the death of an adult child is seen as devastating and tragic. A case is made that this is both limiting and inhuman.

I then explore the impact of the death of a baby on marital intimacy and suggest that the death represents a strain in some relationships as each partner attempts to make sense of their loss. I challenge the concept of gendered emotional responses to loss such that men are tasked with being stoic and women with being vulnerable. I argue that while these dominant discourses provide some explanation as to the difficulties men and women have in coping, they do no not fully explore other important mediating factors such as the presence of surviving siblings in the family. Yet this is critical to understanding varying parental responses to loss and to their sense of identity as a parent. Further, it is this sense of self which is important in exploring ambivalent parental identity and social roles.

In keeping with Giddens (1991), I argue that society continues to 'other' the death of a baby, in that it is viewed as unique, a rare phenomenon, uncommon to the social networks to which we relate. Yet unlike the death of a child, perinatal death is not socially recognised and as a consequence a parents' sense of self and identity is challenged and their grief disenfranchised until that is, they receive recognition for their loss in the form of a sub-culture of bereavement.

For this reason, I conclude by affirming that parental and social responses to perinatal death are complex and multifaceted in that both men and women are exposed to a range of discourses pertaining to the death of their babies and that their expressions and experiences of grief are socially constructed. Such experiences are explored further in relation to health professional discourse and death (Chapter 3) and in light of parental perceptions of health professional responses to their loss (Chapter 7).

The Meaning(s) of the Death of a Child

In chapter 1, it was suggested that the prescriptive format to grief work emphasised a model which could be applied to all bereavement situations. Yet several studies have shown that bereavement through the loss of a son or daughter evokes intense grief reactions and is widely recognised as a severe and difficult form of loss to live with (Klass, 1996; Leon, 2005; Raphael, 1983). The sense of disorder following the loss of a child has also been referred to as an *"amputation of the self"* (Marwitt and Klass, 1996:297). For Schiff (1977:40): *"it is as though parents are not fully alive anymore, they place themselves in the ground when their child has died."* While this does not imply that other losses are less significant, on the contrary they need to be viewed in the context of their meaning. In this respect, the death of a child as it is referred to here is about the loss of a child at any age.

By turning to recent figures about some of these deaths, it is possible to illuminate their prevalence in England and Wales. For example, nearly four thousand children died before they reached their first birthday in 1995. While fewer died between the ages of one and fourteen, the deaths of such children added another two thousand to the mortality figures. Though these ages vary, so do the nature of their deaths including withdrawal from life support, accidental drowning, murders, traffic accidents, illness, disease, suicide (Riches and Dawson, 2000:49). This suggests that the death of a child is far from rare, yet it is argued that modern attitudes towards death may make it unique to the social networks in which we interact. In this context, the meaning of the death of a child is about what the loss represents for parents whether about the loss of an adolescent or infant, it is a grief deeply felt none the less.

The meaning of the death of a child as it is discussed here reflects recent modern attitudes about childhood and that it can somehow be protected. This contrasts with those ideas of childhood in the eighteenth century when it was expected that many children would die (Ariès,1974). Though the death of a child may have represented sadness, for Ariès (1974) it represented a perception of a child as an economic commodity which contributed to the family.

More modern perceptions of 'abnormal' deaths in childhood signifies the transition of children as a commodity that is 'economically useful' to a child in the modern age, that is 'economically priceless' in that they are regarded as a luxury item for which there is no recompense should they die. This reflects the social construction of parenting a 'priceless' childhood in western societies more widely. Indeed, modern attitudes to death make reference to the death of a child in individual social networks as rare and, thus, it appears as something which happens to others.

Yet the loss of a child is such that it *also* needs to be viewed according to a loss of a potential future. In this context, deaths of children after the first four weeks of life are considered separately to those which occur following stillbirth and at neonatal phases, since I argue that the death of a baby at these ages does not receive the same social endorsement or recognition afforded other deaths which occur among other older children.

To this end, I turn to recent figures to illuminate current trends for stillbirth and neonatal death.

Table 1. Stillbirth and Neonatal Death Rates in the UK, 2006

	Rate	Total
Stillbirth	5.3 per 1000 live births	3,987
Neonatal death	3.5 per 1000 live deaths	2,607
		6,594

Office for National Statistics (2006)

The mortality rate per live births in Table 1 demonstrates that for every 1,000 births approximately nine babies die. When seventeen babies are dying each day in the UK, it is for parents at least, a phenomenon which is far from rare. In the case of stillbirth over half are unexplained deaths, which have implications for parents who search for the cause of death as a way of making sense of their loss.

In parents' search for meaning, Klass (1996: 13), refers to an 'empty historical track' in which a biography of the child is crudely disrupted and with it the dreams and hopes of a future. For Klass, parents can be reminded at various junctures what their child would have been doing months and years later. There may also be other poignant anniversaries which have particular relevance to individuals according to their social and cultural orientation. Grief can be long lasting and can stay with parents throughout their life time. These experiences may be subjected to a social hierarchy of grief since the death of the child does not fall within the accepted age range of what is deemed a tragic child death, for example, perinatal death (Rando, 1991).

For Emery (1990: 423): *"There has been a tendency to look upon bereavement as a profit and loss account, the more you have, if you lose it the greater the loss – a sort of love balance."* Emery is referring to an understanding of the meaning of the loss of a child which is in keeping with the evolutionary psychology perspective. Indeed, for Wright: *"Just as a horse breeder is more disappointed by the death of a thoroughbred the day before its first race than the day after its birth, a parent should be more heartbroken by the death of an adolescent than by the death of an infant. Both the adolescent and the mature racehorse are assets on the brink of bringing rewards, and in both cases it will take much time and effort, starting from scratch, to get another asset to that point."* (1994:174)

Wright suggests that children who vary in age from one another will also vary in terms of the time and effort that has been placed in rearing them and in terms of their potential for producing future generations. It follows from this view that a greater sense of loss and pain is felt for an adolescent who has died than the death of a baby, since the former has received the greatest number of invested years compared to that of an infant at twelve months of age or less. Furthermore, an adolescent has a greater chance of producing offspring since as human evolutionary history suggests, a one year old has had a much lesser chance of survival (Archer, 1999:151).

Other authors (Littlefield and Rushton, 1986) have attempted to apply evolutionary principles in their research pertaining to grief. They hypothesised that parents would experience a greater intensity of grief for the death of older children compared to parents whose child has died at younger ages, in particular, in infancy. However, the findings of both studies suggest that there was no association found between the age of the child when they died and the intensity of grief experienced by parents.

The age to investment loss equation (as applied by the evolutionary psychology thesis) fails to consider the fact that there is no direct line which emanates from our genes to explain why certain behaviours such as grief are acted out in response to life events (death).

It can be argued that the severity of grief experienced by individuals corresponds to the closeness and attachment of personal relationships (Archer, 2001:158). De Vries et al's (1994:52), findings from narratives on loss from interviews with bereaved parents further challenges the evolutionary psychology thesis. They noted that 'younger' parents viewed 'older' parents as at least having had more years with their child, while they had none or some and were denied the hope of a future potential relationship with their child. Conversely, the older parents felt not only the loss of a child and for some a friend, but also the emotional investment they had placed in the relationship. They further suggested that an effective coping strategy would be to have another child since this would reinstate the role of a parent. However for others (Ashurst and Hall, 1989) a dead child cannot be replaced and no other child can be a substitute for one that has been loved and lost.

It is useful to be reminded of the discussion in Chapter 1, about Freud's despair following his experience of significant deaths in his life. Freud's solemnity is important since it is reflective of parents' accounts of subsequent children in Chapter 7 and their continued feelings of grief for the baby who has died. It is, as with Freud, a grief work which can never be completed.

Freud experienced the death of a child in adulthood, which for some parents may exacerbate the losses already experienced as an ageing person, namely social status, job, and friends. It is suggested that these losses are not confined to 'older' or retired parents, they can occur among parents whose child has died as a result of stillbirth and neonatal death.

Stillbirth and neonatal death evokes a bereavement response which is so profound it has drawn the attention of several researchers (Benfield et al, 1978; Giles, 1970; Kavanaugh, 1997). While recognised as just like any other death, the death of a child in infancy represents a loss of a significant other, a loss of part of the self, and the hopes and dreams for the future. It may also evoke fear - the loss of hope of being able to bear children (O'Leary, 2009). Despite the attention given by these researchers as to the uniqueness of infant death, the main body of literature pertaining to perinatal loss primarily focuses on the impact on parents who experience the death of their stillborn infants.

Few studies exist which account for the uniqueness of the grief which follows the death of a neonatal baby in particular, in the special care baby unit when the death of their baby occurs as a result of withdrawal from life support (Armentrout, 2005). Parents' experiences on the neonatal ward have been underrepresented due to a lack of sociological research and an over emphasis in the medical literature to define such experience according to professional perspectives. It is useful to consider the meaning of the death of a baby in a way in which other sociological writers (Rando, 1991:9) have framed it and where the baby is viewed as the very antithesis of death.

The Meaning(s) of the Death of a Baby

"An umbilical cord is nature's ventilator and a whole lot more. She was flesh of our flesh and to say she was never born is to deny our very own existence." (Don, 2005: 72)

"The Death of a baby, whether at birth or in the weeks or months immediately afterwards, is no less a death than any other....It is certainly different, but it is not a lesser event." (Kohner and Henley, 1997: xi)

The last two decades have witnessed a proliferation of research that addresses perinatal loss and bereavement (Caelli et al, 2002:366; Condon, 1986; Forrest et al, 1982; Turton et al, 2001) in particular the emotional consequences experienced by parents following stillbirth and neonatal death. Parents, particularly mothers, have reportedly expressed guilt, remorse, anger, anxiety, rage, fear, resentment, jealousy, envy, loneliness, and sorrow (Hughes and Riches, 2003; Peppers and Knapp, 1980). While writers such as Hughes and Riches (2003:112) suggest that parents experiencing the death of their baby can expect an improvement in their grief within six months after the death, this is an assumption widely challenged (Forrest et al, 1982; Hughes et al, 1999; Rando, 1991; Turton, et al, 2001). Men and women may not only grieve for long periods of time but may in fact continue to grieve for the rest of their lives, even if with effort and difficulty they resume daily activities (Schwab, 1992). It is suggested that this experience is challenging for parents since it is a grief which is not culturally sanctioned.

This is in keeping with Kellner and Lake (1990) who argue that the death of a baby represents a *forgotten grief* since stillbirth is seldom acknowledged in western culture; people tend to find it difficult to appreciate the existence of a stillborn baby as a person, especially if they have not seen the child. While they may ponder over the events, there may be little appreciation of the emotional impact of the death.

Despite the meaning given to the baby by the parents, the birth and death is conflated as though one cancels out the other in the process of *giving birth to death* (Layne, 2003:177). It is an experience, which represents a tragedy least expected by many men and women, yet reflects a taken for granted way of thinking about pregnancy more widely.

The Taken for Granted Pregnancy

The feminist writer Linda Layne (2003:174) argues that a pregnancy which ends in stillbirth or neonatal death is itself tragic, yet the outcome is devastatingly worse than would-be parents anticipated. For Layne, the loss is shocking since events did not turn out as expected and the depth of the irony is in large part owed to what one might expect to happen (e.g. a healthy baby) to what actually happens which is a death.

For Layne (2003:175), the death of a baby can be experienced as an unthinkable and devastating deviation from the natural, the normal, biological and social progression that pregnancies are expected to entail and have come to be understood in the medical model terms of foetal development. Though this exposes taken for granted ideas about pregnancy and birth more widely, Layne fails to note varying pregnant narratives. For example, stillbirths follow from deaths which are expected and unexpected occurring as they do in utero (in the womb), during labour, soon after and as a result of abnormalities. What exacerbates the sense of loss is not irony, but the expectations that biomedicine and modern technology can now fix any problems associated with the body including pregnancy and birth. The social transformation from would-be parents, to the parents of a dead baby is consequential since men and women lose their 'innocence' about pregnancy and birth. Indeed, parents' life narratives can become punctuated by the death, such that other experiences come to be understood as having occurred either before or after this event.

Such trauma is complicated further by the notion that stillbirth or neonatal death represents nothing more *than a disappointment* (Kirkley-Best, 1981:421). Further, that there is an assumed greater investment in the infant by the mother than the father which brings about a closer emotional bond with the unborn baby and their mother. This perspective supposes that fathers are viewed as having little or no attachment to the baby since the presence of the *biological-tactile* relationship experienced by the mother cannot exist for the father, and, thus, their entitlement to grief is reduced (Archer, 1999:156).

Several authors (Kirkley-Best 1981; Kirkley-Best and Kellner, 1982) have challenged these assumptions and argued that while attachment may not exist in its biological form, fathers develop cognitive attachments to the baby in the same way as mothers.

An accurate account of any gender differences is problematic given the number of studies and articles which focus on the parent at the individual level and aim to compare and contrast grief responses. This is despite the fact that the majority of parents will have been living together at the time of loss and need to be viewed in the context of their relationship to each other. To this end I consider gendered emotional responses to loss since it will be shown in proceeding chapters that the response of each parent to their spouse mediates their experience of grief in the relationship.

Gendered Emotional Responses to Grief

> *"Societal norms seem to promote an aesthetic standard of the right way to grieve, rather than an appreciation of the obvious: that people are different, as are their attachments to their newborn and unborn children and the manner and degree to which they mourn their dead babies."* (Leon, 1992:8)

The emotional response to bereavement has received widespread attention particularly since the 1950s, yet the gendered response to grief following stillbirth and neonatal death and the way in which emotion is influenced remains unclear. This is despite the assertions of sociologists Riches and Dawson (1997:55), that grief is a socially and culturally constructed entity. This suggests that the reasons why open expression and reaction is seen to differ between men and women are because of the influence of gender structured patterns of emotional response. However, it is also suggested that gender is not only the 'objective' aspect of human experience, it is also a dimension of the internal, subjective experience. From this perspective, gender not only shapes how women and men conduct themselves following loss, but also how social institutions mediate the subjective experience of grief at the cognitive and affective level (Thompson, 1997: 78).

For sociologists such as Thompson (1997), men's grief responses can be viewed as different from women's since the way men respond to loss can be defined according to a division of discursive labour. For example, women may look to their emotional and expressive knowledge to address grief and adjustment following loss. Thus, their expression of grief is likely to be informed by their life experiences of emotional discourses. Men's responses to loss are, thus, explained as a joint management of the marital emotional expression of supporting a partner or wife and of their organisation and supervision around the time of the death (funeral). Men may be informed by discourses which characterise the public, social and cultural expression of grief.

Yet the changing economic and social role of men and women underpins the debate about re-evaluating assumptions which emphasise the link between the women as belonging to the private sphere (weeping at home) and the men to the public domain (organising the public funeral).

What is suggested is that the resources available to men and women following loss may well be gendered, yet women's increasing economic activity and the impact of feminism on men may expose both men and women to a range of discourses pertaining to the death of a baby, which includes being exposed to other discourses in society. For example, Radley (1989), argues that emotional responses to events are managed by creating an 'illness identity', which is constructed mainly out of conversations between marital partnerships, which in itself is a marital discourse drawing upon wider discourses of gender, class, and medicine.

Radley's idea about differing emotional responses is based primarily upon Durkheim's distinction of mechanistic and organic social relationships. Radley (1989), applied this notion to patients from various social classes who experienced heart disease. He noted that patients defined as middle class had a tendency to view their illness as an experience to be managed in contrast to 'working class' patients who viewed their experience of heart disease with fatalism.

Following Radley's study, and later Douglas and Calvez' (1990) perceptions of risk from HIV, Riches and Dawson (1997:53) conducted a sociological study and explored emotional responses to grief in their study of parents following the death of a child. Their findings suggest that the type of social support provided by family, friends, and colleagues to parents mediated their experience of grief and sense of self. While some parents responded that family and friends often failed to recognise how devastating the death of their child is, others acknowledged their loss, thereby legitimising their grief.

As parents attempted to find meaning, there was for some, a renewed strength in their relationship with their husband or wife which was observed by Riches and Dawson as a sense–making discourse within intimate relationships.

This discussion on gendered emotional responses to loss exposes cultural beliefs about gender more widely. For Thompson (1997), gender stereotypes carry descriptive information about how men and women are culturally assumed to be and prescriptive information about how they should respond to situations. A violation of this prescriptive gender expectation provokes a negative backlash unless that is; responses are legitimated in particular situations. This can occur in situations where gender is not particularly salient such as in all female or male groups. In the context of relationships does not the level of marital intimacy play a part? As Rubin (2007:319) notes, the common wisdom is that women want intimacy and men resist it. This in part explains perceived differing responses to loss by men and women in their marital relationships with one another. In turning to marital intimacy, the extent to which the death of a child impacts more widely on couples is explored.

Marital Intimacy

The loss of a child has reportedly produced a great deal of strain in marital intimacy somehow significant enough to result in permanent separation or divorce (Lang et al, 1996, Najman et al, 1993). While there is scant literature as to the effect on partnerships (parents who are unmarried), studies pertaining to the effect on a marriage following loss estimate that serious marital difficulties are experienced by as many as 80 percent of bereaved couples within a few months of a loss of a baby (SANDS, 2009:10). Increased communication difficulties, emotional isolation and mutual frustration between couples are reported, with much of the tension assumed to relate to differences in grieving patterns (Littlewood, et al, 1991; Schwab, 1992).

The significance of the variance of distress expressed by each parent in the relationship has been explained as incongruent grieving, in that it is assumed one partner is less affected by the death (Peppers and Knapp, 1980). Other authors (Wallerstedt and Higgins, 1996), suggest that the presence of tension in a relationship is attributable to the role each parent is socialised into in that the father may feel the need to be stoic, organised and strong, and the mother as a result may view the father as uncaring and even cold. Conversely, the father may feel the mother's need to be open and emotional as intense.

While the gendered images of the bereaved following the loss of a child provide some explanation as to varying grief responses, Riches and Dawson (1997:52-53) report exceptions to this rule.

In their study of parental responses to the death of the child, Riches and Dawson found that while most fathers appeared to be stoic and attempted to support their wives, there were men among the sample who grieved as openly as the mothers. Further, while mothers reported recurring feelings of despair and distress and expressed them openly, they were re--engaged in fulltime work or other activities relatively soon after their bereavement, and appeared to reveal coping styles which are usually associated with men. Of note is that variations in respondents' grief responses appeared to be associated with the availability of a supportive social network. Upon this basis it is the nature of the marriage which significantly mediates grief responses. This is in keeping with other authors (Berger and Kellner, 1964; Deal et al, 1992) who attest that marriage is about a continuous negotiation of mutual understandings about the world. This suggests that the death of a child represents a severe challenge to a parents' ability to agree on the meaning of the loss to one another.

While several authors have suggested that parents experience marital difficulties following the loss of a child, others (Rando, 1991; Lang and Gottlieb, 1996) suggest that couples experience a change in their bond to one another in addition to new estrangements due to individual responses within marriage to that loss and it is this which creates communication difficulties, misunderstandings, and tension in a relationship (Peppers and Knapp, 1980; Rando, 1991; Schwab, 1992).

Much of the evidence concerning intra couple distress is inconclusive given the relatively small sample sizes and the paucity of longitudinal data to assess changing needs of parents over time. Yet the literature on gendered responses to loss and marital intimacy overwhelmingly suggests a widening rift in the relationship following a death and that as a consequence parents may feel isolated at a time when they need support the most (Caelli et al, 2002). This is interesting given the propensity of the marital intimacy literature to emphasise negativity in a relationship compared to the closeness in the bond it may bring.

The marital intimacy literature as with the psychological emphasises 'typical' gendered responses to loss, which, it is argued, are not entirely useful when research suggests that these distinctions become blurred. These gender distinctions are so firmly fixed and built into psychological thought that they are seen as an exogenous, scientific truth. Though it can be seen that intimacy is difficult in some relationships it represents a paradox. Since in this emotionality and expressivity, men particularly return to their childhood experiences with their mother (Rubin, 2007:323). Though this represents the power of experiences with a mother, it is these early experiences and the man's need to learn to resist and repress them which acts as the conduit to a sense of ambivalence to emotionality, which is perceived as resistance in relationships.

Thus, gender distinctions may be a less useful variable in examining the existence of marital tension and responses to grief following the death of a baby. Rather, there are few discourses which parents can refer to in their grief other than those which focus upon the abnormality of a death in infancy. Moreover, the social expectations of motherhood place strong definitions about the situation onto the mother who is bereaved and much less so upon the father. A more useful way to consider the social factors and influences which mediate men and women's responses to loss is to explore how the death of a baby changes a sense of self and identity.

The Meaning of Motherhood and Fatherhood

> *"We must never forget that we may also find meaning in life even when confronted with a hopeless situation, when facing a fate that cannot be changed. For what then matters is to bear witness to the uniquely human potential...when we are no longer able to change a situation, we are challenged to change ourselves."* (Frankl, 2006:112)

There has been a tendency to consider the pathological responses to loss following the death of a baby at the expense of articulating the reasons why the impact is more complex than it appears. Sociological researchers such as Riches and Dawson (1997), have focused upon how such a loss changes a parent's identity and sense of self. There are many definitions of the concept of self. For Silverman (2000:45) the self is the ability to process and connect experiences, to direct behaviour, to know who the individual is and what they are doing. This sense of self changes when we differentiate ourselves from those of others and how others are included in our lives. The development of the self is the result of relationship with others. Piaget (quoted in Youniss, 1980) wrote: *"There are no such things as isolated individuals. There are only relations. There is no sense of self outside relations because the self can only know itself in reference to other selves."*(1980:4) When death occurs the self that was formed by the relationship to the deceased is lost. Cote-Arsenault (2003: 282), suggests that there is no child to nurture and, thus, society does not acknowledge the mother or father as a parent to that particular child. Familial roles, then, provide the core constructs of our identity, and can serve as a principal source of who we are. Representational systems are a part of culture since culture includes a way of making sense of our lives. Culture is not simply reflecting meanings, it creates them.

The concern here is with meanings and how they are produced. In the context of motherhood, the body for Woodward (2003:19) is more than a maternal and biological carrier: it comes to be a site which is inscribed by culture and society and it is this which provides meaning.

In this respect, motherhood is an identity which is subject to assumptions about taken for granted pregnancies and birth in popular discourse and to the plethora of techniques through which meanings are derived about being a mother. This represents a paradox for women following stillbirth and neonatal death since when is a parent, a parent? On the one hand, the physicality of pregnancy signifies a status as 'expectant parent' while the physical work of labour has delivered a child that has died or soon will.

In contemporary western culture, notions of motherhood and bereaved parent status are particularly ambiguous. For Woodward (2003:18), motherhood is subject to contested and idealised representations, through the symbolic regimes which produce meanings about the experience. Similarly, Layne (2003) considers the act of gift giving in post birthing encounters and congratulatory symbols of cards and flowers which help to mark the new status of mother. The point for Layne is that in situations of loss there is limited socially ritualistic opportunity to conduct symbolic acts since it is deemed inappropriate. Yet ideas about motherhood are critical to understanding women's sense of ambivalent status following loss.

Traditional representations of motherhood are closely aligned to a historical trajectory of the 1950s stay-at-home mum, giving way to the 'having it all – career and family' mum of the latter part of the twentieth century and to the 'celebrity mums' represented more recently in popular magazines. Though these representations of mothering seem to confer a certain identity, social and technological developments demand a greater clarity. What of surrogacy, step-parenting, egg donor mother, adoptive mother and a whole other range of ways of being a mother? Moreover, these ideas are contested in court rooms and debated in the media in terms of ownership and who has the 'right' to be a mother whether as a lesbian, or an older woman, or when an adolescent. The point is that motherhood is assumed to form part of the natural biographical trajectory of women's lives. It represents a populist taken for granted plot to women's lives which end up as chaotic narratives of a wrecked part of life when a child dies.

66

This wreckage is a direct response to ambivalent identity construction, a key element of which is subjective reality. Like all subjective reality it stands in dialectical relationship with society (Berger and Luckman, 1966:173). To this end, it can be seen that identity is formed by social and cultural processes. The problem with this wisdom however is that there are sources of discrepancy between what is felt by women following loss and the feeling rules which society ascribes these situations (which are in themselves ambivalent), which provide for non-normative role transitions. These changes represent ambiguity precisely because it is not known what the identity of such women is. Consequently, women's reproductive biographies represent narratives which are both wrecked and chaotic in their telling. Thus, meaning comes to be represented by interruption, disruption and ambiguity. This extends to ideas about fatherhood and the question when does a man become a father.

For decades, fatherhood has been subject to much public debate concerning 'traditional' versus the 'new' model of fathering (Freeman, 2003:33). Though the traditional father implies paternal deference while the 'new' father is symbolic of more equal parenting in relationships, they represent an ideological crisis which has been politicized nonetheless. For Freeman (2003:34), it follows that the current crisis in defining the meaning of fatherhood is rooted in wider, cultural, economic and social processes.

While this represents ideas more widely about conceptions of good fathering versus bad male parenting, it points to the diversification of fathering identity roles within the family and in society (stepfather, biological father, sperm donor, adoptive father). Thus, the presentation of self as the father in itself invariably draws upon a pool of pre-established discourses within wider society and in specific social contexts.

Similarly, people are placed by others (relatives, colleagues, and friends) in discursive interactions as particular individuals (Lupton and Barclay, 1997:9). It can be seen that an aspect to describing the self is exploring the means by which they experience and define themselves.

As previously noted, fatherhood is a phenomenon subject to competing discourses which frame and give meaning to identity and are at the site of the struggle in claiming fatherhood following loss. In this respect, bereaved men are subject to similar role ambivalences as grieving women following the deaths of their babies. This does not deny the capacity of these different bodies in these experiences, on the contrary, it shapes the type of participation men and women have in relation to pregnancy and birth more widely. The point is that while these anatomical differences are retained in this discussion concerning identity, the contingent nature of knowledge and experience of reality recognises that the meanings given to these are socially constructed and mediated in encounters with others. As men and women make sense of experience and reconstruct their accounts of loss, they do so from their embodied position in the social world (Miller, 2005:113).

Having explored the complexities in defining notions of motherhood and fatherhood following loss, it is to surviving siblings I now turn to discuss some of the ways children mediate parent's experiences.

Surviving Siblings

Cecil, (1996), suggests that women who have children prior to their loss experience less anxiety compared to women who were childless who experienced greater distress. Referred to as the *forgotten mourners* (Hindmarch, 1995:37), bereaved brothers and sisters have received less attention from researchers interested in bereavement and as a consequence there is a paucity of literature about the impact upon the parent to child relationship and how this influences responses to loss in the family. While there are some texts about childhood bereavement, few are based upon studies with consistent findings (Dent and Stewart, 2004:72).

For writers about childhood bereavement such as Dent and Stewart (2004), changes in intimacy in the surviving child–maternal relationship can affect up to eighty percent of families where the youngest member (a baby) dies. For example, increased aggressiveness features highly since the child blames the mother for the death of the child and may even encourage the mother to have 'another' baby to avoid repeating the same 'mistake'.

Where parents may long for a baby, subsequent pregnancies and births can be an anxiety–ridden experience for most parents (Kirkley-Best, 1981 and DeVries et al, 1994). Further, the next baby born alive may be viewed as a replacement vehicle for the child that died and consequently feel unable to live up to the expectations of its parents (Kirkley-Best, 1981 and DeVries etal, 1994). Indeed for Condon (1986) the deceased baby represents:*"a recipient par excellence of projected aspects of the spouse. In addition, its representation is coloured by the woman's own and society's beliefs and myths about pregnancy and babies"* (1986:89). It is the unique relationship with the baby who has died that poignantly and powerfully differentiates the loss in stillbirth and neonatal death from that of other bereavements within the family and the need for more specialized support for the family and surviving children.

Our knowledge of the perspectives of bereaved siblings is limited so that there is a need for understanding both the short and life-long effects and some of the ways familial responses to loss mediate individual members' bereavement experiences. While this is a subject that requires a greater amount of research, it is limited in scope within this thesis to parents' experiences. This discussion about surviving siblings, though brief, represents a way to explain the extent to which men and women mourn their losses. For Klass (1996): *"Parenting is a permanent change in the individual. A person never gets over being a parent. Parental bereavement is also a permanent condition. The bereaved parent, after a time, will cease showing the medical symptoms of grief, but the parent does not "get over" the death of the child."* (1996:178)

69

Following research with mothers following the loss of a baby, Layne (2003) describes the status of parent of a deceased baby as 'liminal' (an in between state). In this sense, parents feel that they are parents (they have conceived and birthed) yet are no longer parenting the child. Given this disjunction parents seek to continue their attachments with the baby. There is evidence by Rubin (1984) to suggest that women experience a continuing relationship with their baby sometimes for years following the death. What is important in Rubin's research is that it distinguishes between the adjustment required in relation to the external reality of the loss and the nature of the ongoing relationship which is internally represented.

For Marris (1991), attachment can be interwoven with meaning since the attachments we make are the first and most crucial relationships by which we learn to organise meaning. Grief is therefore, a response to the loss that fundamentally challenges the purpose of life and represents an existential dilemma.

For example, De Frain et al's (1990-1) study of 850 family members who had been affected by perinatal death kept asking: 'Why did this happen' and 'Why me?' These responses severely test the frameworks of meaning some individuals may adopt to interpret their experiences of the world, which have variously been referred to as a 'socially constructed reality' (Berger and Luckman, 1966), and a 'prior meaning structure' (Braun and Berg, 1994). As Talbot (1997) explains: *"In our world of everyday life, we each have access to our own personal reservoir of socially derived knowledge. This knowledge consists of clear, consistent and unquestionably valid 'knowledge about' people, places, and things, knowledge which has been tested and passed onto us by others, and which explains the what, how and why of social life....* (1997:49) This way of thinking about life and the world is continuously shifting as these interpretations are shared allowing individuals to act in predictable concert with one another. It can be seen that when these interpretations are not shared, conflict arises.

A number of sociological writers (Giddens, 1991; Handley, 1991; Mellor and Schilling, 1993) argue that the internal working models acquired by individuals are inadequate for preparing them for death. By drawing upon the work of Giddens (1991), it can be seen that part of parents' confusion stems from their great sense of responsibility for protecting their children from harm whilst having a sense of trust in the world. Upon the death of a baby, the dissonance between the interpretation of the event and the prevailing concept that the world is benevolent and predictable shatters these implicit assumptions and leads to a sense of disorientation. Giddens argues that our natural attitude to life keeps away questions about our mortal selves, in the sense that if death happens at all, it happens to others. It is this which provides a safe way of getting answers to frameworks of existence which are emotional.

Thus, individuals tend to take for granted their everyday activities and their way of thinking about the world because it remains unchallenged. Yet they are in no way grounded by the interactional conventions they observe in society nor the contradictions of the dominant discourses of the culture, for example medicine and its heroic efforts to save lives yet its inability (at times) to avert the death of a baby, such that these deaths are regarded as extraordinary. Indeed, people's practical consciousness together with the daily routines they live help to contain such anxieties about death primarily because of the social stability they imply and also for their role in organizing an 'as if' way of thinking in relation to what Giddens refers to as existential issues. As he explains: *"On the other side of what might appear to be quite trivial aspects of day to day action and discourse, chaos lurks. And this chaos is not just disorganization, but the loss of a sense of the very reality of things and of other persons."* (Giddens, 1991:36) This supports the notion that the internal working models employed by most individuals in modern societies are inadequate for preparing them for making sense of a child death.

The point to stress here is that the death of a child challenges not only the deepest assumptions about life and the world for the bereaved parent, but threatens others who would prefer not to contemplate their own or their child's mortality. Arguably, few people want to know what the death of a child is like, since such insight may not only be terrifying but bring about the realisation that our families, work and lives are fragile and temporary. Yet the death of a baby is not rare; it may be relatively unfamiliar in people's social networks but in modern societies, attitudes towards the death may make it feel as though it is a unique phenomenon. It is therefore argued that contemporary social responses to death and the bereaved necessitate a shared framework of reality and of truly knowing such experience which explains why some people seek the help of a support group, the web and alternative resources.

Moreover, published accounts of loss in the literature suggest that both men and women have employed this way of expressing grief and finding meaning. This further suggests that men and women want to continue to talk and make reference to their baby, and it is these resources (book, web or group) which provide reassurance (Aho et al, 2009). Yet it is this knowledge which to a large extent has yet to be transferred to the death studies debate within sociology.

Conclusion

Before turning to the sociology of emotions and the medical discourse of emotions in relation to perinatal loss in Chapter 3, it is useful to reflect upon the main themes in relation to grief and loss and the death of a child. It was acknowledged that the latter was a difficult form of loss to live with, yet in the evolutionary psychology view of life deaths of adolescents were seen as more distressing than the deaths of infants. Despite this inhumane reference to the death of younger children, this was a notion that could not stand in light of contrary research, yet was useful in so far as to reflect the tendency of psychology to marginalise other important social influences.

By employing sociological concepts, it was shown that there was a tendency towards descriptive and symptomatic language when trying to explain varying gendered emotional responses to loss in the perinatal literature. Rather, it was sociologically proffered that men's experience and expression of grief differed yet was not deficient to that of women. It was argued that the resources available to parents after loss may be gendered, yet women's increasing economic activity and the impact of feminism on men may expose both men and women to a range of discourses pertaining to the death of a baby, which includes being exposed to other discourses in society. While this provided some explanation for varying experiences and responses to loss, I argued that there were other important mediating factors which need to be explored in light of parents' grief, in particular the influence of surviving siblings.

This is important to the debate about parents' ambivalent social status following loss. I argued that while parenting surviving children denoted a status, it was unable to fulfil that of being a parent to the child who had died, since the death was not socially recognised. Consequently, parents continue to grieve for a loss which is disenfranchised, until they seek membership of a sub-culture of bereavement to explore the meaning of the death of their child. I pointed to the contradiction in this by arguing that the death of an infant is far from rare, yet in contemporary society attitudes towards death render it abnormal which makes it a unique experience for bereaved parents. This in part relates to society's unquestioning faith in the ability of medicine to avert death which leads to confusion.

Yet society's response to the death of a child can be viewed as a cultural product which can be found in public discourses. Thus, culture provides the content of grieving while social support systems and relationships both facilitate and constrain responses to loss. It is complex, not least because the death of a child is viewed as an unimaginable event, difficult to contemplate and as such becomes 'othered' and even denied.

While perinatal death may indeed be unusual and uncommon in people's social network, it is nonetheless an event which is experienced by individuals in society. These individuals are left to find meaning as there is little in the way of a script to define ways to respond to parents which are supportive and conducive to handling their loss.

To this end I maintain that men and women's experiences are mediated by the cultural experience of death and its expression which is socially constructed. Grief is therefore a cultural product as well as a psychological response mediated by social relations.

These ideas are considered further in the next chapter, which explores health professional responses to the death of a baby and the discourses which inform their practice.

CHAPTER 3. The Sociology of Emotions and the Medical Discourse of Emotions

> "Emotion is a sense that tells about the self-relevance of reality. We infer from it what we must have wanted or expected or how we must have been perceiving the world. Emotion is one way to discover a buried perspective on matters, especially when other ways of locating ourselves are in bad repair." (Hochschild, 2003:85)

Introduction

Previous chapters explored multidisciplinary approaches to understanding death, ritual and mourning in society (Chapter 1), and the existing literature about grief and loss following the death of a child (Chapter 2). It has been argued that the medical discourse in relation to death, dying and grief represents a discursive framework about a form of knowledge. In this context, medicine provides a way in which to perceive health and illness such that it has become a dominant discourse in understanding social life and meaning in society. One of the features of the medical profession in modern Britain is the integral role played by doctors and nurses in the management of death and dying.

In this chapter I consider representations of professional discourse in the context of emotionality and expressivity within medical encounters to explain varying professional approaches to perinatal loss in hospital (Chapter 7). In so doing, I explore the sociology of emotions which has attracted a number of classical and contemporary theorists including the oft cited researches of Hochschild's (2003) 'emotional management' thesis, first published in 1983. This body of knowledge is considered in light of the biology versus society debate on emotions in which the organismic model compares to the social constructionist and interactional orientations. Completing these analyses are phenomenological approaches which suggest that the ontological basis of self is borne of sensory experience. It will be shown that emotions are necessarily embodied and mediated by the individual, social and political in medical encounters.

A case is made that emotionality within medicine represents an element of work which is consequential and subject to the 'feeling rules' of the 'corporate structure.' This sense of corporeality within maternity and neonatal units is dependent upon a level of coherency in professional working practices. I argue that this is lacking and in part explains varying professional approaches to the perinatal loss encounter. It therefore follows that a discussion of the limitations of more recent policies and guidelines proposed by the voluntary sector (SANDS) is considered in light of the emotion work performed in medical encounters. By drawing on the social interactional and organismic approach of Hochschild, it will be shown that emotions represent an aspect of work which is expected, yet not supported in medical training. This reflects a medical discourse more widely, the foundation of which rests upon a Cartesian, Western, scientific model of emotion. This discussion is foregrounded by an examination of the socio-political aspects of perinatal death. I consider legislation in defining foetal personhood and, thus, parental identity which, I argue informs social and medical practice.

I conclude by arguing that emotions are not only central to debates in mainstream sociological theory, they are critical to an understanding of experience more widely in society. Emotions are embodied experiences and ones which involve active engagement with the world, culture and the self.

Organismic and Social Interactional Models of Emotion

Dismissed as 'irrational', private and inner sensations, emotions represent the very antithesis of objectivity and wisdom in dominant, Western, scientific and social thought (Williams and Bendelow, 1996). This dualism of reason/emotion, mind versus body and nature or culture, can be found in the modern views of Descartes (1637/1985): *'Cogito, ergo sum'* – I think therefore I am. In his *Discourse on Method*, Descartes, is able to 'think away everything' about himself, since the mind and body are separate entities, simply a part of the external world.

76

In his I *have* a body, I never *am* my body, the materiality of his body is not part of his quintessential self, it is but a spatial extension. This dualism of mind to the body for Descartes was about subject and object, mind and matter, observer and observed. This view of disembodiment is central to divisions within sociological discussions about emotions. Included in these is the micro/macro, quantitative/qualitative, biosocial versus the social constructionist perspectives (Harré, 1991; McCarthy and Doyle, 1989). Other sociological interests regarding emotions can be found within gender analysis and the political economy of emotions (Kemper, 1990). Within these debates, approaches to emotion are conceptualised according to organismic, social constructionist and interactionist perspectives.

The organismic models of emotion can be found in the works of Darwin (1872/1955), Freud (1917/1973) and James and Lange (1922) and defined mainly as a biological process. Where emotion (affect) is libidinal discharge for Freud, for Darwin it is instinct, and for James and Lange emotion is the perception of a biological process. By the focus on instinct and energy, these theorists postulate an emotion which is similarly experienced by all people.

Where emotions are but a biological process for these theorists, interactionists such as Goffman (1959, 1967) are more concerned with the meaning that these psychological processes provide. The focus on emotion as 'motored by instinct' suggests that the way in which emotion is labelled or managed or indeed expressed is of less interest to the organismic theorists. Here, emotion is presumed to be introspective, a process which is passive and lacking in power.

Interactionists question the prior existence of emotions in so much as they are part of the creation of that emerging experience. Where emotion is open ended for interactionists, for organismic theorists it is fixed. The organismic focus on emotion which is instinctual lies at the juncture of its interest in the origins of emotion.

While of little interest to interactionists, these origins to emotion can be traced back to childhood for Freud and to their phylogenetic origin for Darwin.

This focus on origin is diverted in the interactional model towards a focus on emotion as differentiating between social groups. For these theorists, social factors impinge on the formation of these emotions by codification, management and expression.

Darwin's classic book, *The Expression of Emotions in Man and Animals* (1872/1955), proffers a model of emotions for other theorists. In so doing, emotionality and expressivity (e.g. gestures and displays) are explored rather than their subjective meanings. For Darwin, these displays form part of his evolutionary thesis in that they were acquired in pre-historic ages and continued as 'serviceable associated habits'. These useful gestures, while originally linked to actions (*manqué*) can be found when expressing rage where the 'baring of teeth' is a vestige of the once immediate act of biting. Similarly, expressing disgust is the vestige of what was once the act of 'regurgitating a noxious thing' (Hochschild, 2003:217). Darwin's model of emotion, then, is a theory about gestures which are instinctual, but are they universal or culturally specific? For Darwin, they remained universal and innate, a conclusion shared by other theorists (Ekman et al, 1972), and those who have argued that they are modelled from language and, thus, culturally variable (Birdwhistell, 1970; Rosenthal, 2003). However, what Darwin's theory lacked was the concept of emotion as a subjective experience which is impinged upon by social factors.

If for Darwin emotion is instinctual gesture, and for Freud, the manifestation of a damned-up libido, for James it is the mind's response to instinctual visceral changes. As James and Lange (1922) explain in their book *Principles of Psychology*: "......*bodily changes follow directly the perception of the exciting fact and that our feeling of the same changes as they occur is the emotion.*" (cited in Hochschild, 2003:220)

In equating emotion with bodily change, it follows that different emotions will be accompanied by different bodily states. While the interactional model acknowledges the biology of emotion, it, questions the organismic presumption that social factors enter prior to and following these processes. For the interactionists then, it is the way these social factors interact during the experience of emotion which is important. Moreover, these emotions can be seen to vary socially and cross-culturally in terms of their meaning, experience and expression, and are therefore social and cultural constructions.

While few sociological theories dispute the biological substrate in emotions, social constructionists emphasise the social compared to the physiological source of emotions. In this respect, emotions are social and cultural constructions, which while they vary from culture to culture in terms of their meaning, are socially constructed none the less.

For McCarthy and Doyle (1989:57), emotions cannot be explained by organism but instead viewed in relation to the conscious actions, experiences and relation of selves. Emotions are not inside bodies, they are actions which are placed in our social world and constituted by and sustained by social group processes (Williams and Bendelow, 1996).

For Harré (1991), there are ways of acting and feeling within a social and moral order where opinions are displayed in appropriate ways. As Harré explains: *"To be angry is to have taken on the angry role on a particular occasion as the expression of a moral position...... The bodily feeling is often the somatic expression to oneself of the taking of a moral standpoint."* (1991:142-3) Concluding these works are the rules, in which social and emotional actions are critically evaluated, maintained or altered (Harré, 1991:13). Within this framework, emotions are at best peripheral emerging as phenomena according to the social and cultural milieu to which they belong.

Thus, any physiological changes which accompany these emotions are not explained. This more Goffmanesque consideration of emotional management is central to Collins's (1990) ideas concerning the way micro-interactional processes relate to socio structural issues of order and conflict.

For Collins, social order (a central process of macro sociology) is dependent upon the micro level of emotions. It is maintained at the micro level of emotions through the rituals and emotional exchanges which emerge from them. These micro/macro mediations of emotions can be seen to maintain such order with sentiments which deploy negative sentiments towards those with opposing social values. Similarly, for Turner (2007): *"Societies are ultimately held together by the positive emotions that people feel toward social structures and culture; and, conversely, societies can be torn apart and changed by the arousal of both negative and positive emotions."* (2007:179). For Turner, emotions emerge at the micro level of social reality which, under certain conditions generate the pressure for stasis or change within a social structure.

In keeping with the idea of co-variance between social structures, interactions and emerging emotions, Kemper's (1990) more positivist stance suggests a process of emotion which can be predicted. For Kemper it follows that interactions based on power and status generate emotions. Within social situations, individuals possess relative power (authority) and the ability to tell others what to do (status). This is not a status which is seen as a position within a structure but as an honour, a sign of prestige. This status relates to the giving and receiving of deference. When people have power they experience positive emotions such as satisfaction, security and confidence. When they don't, emotions are framed in a negative light and experienced as anxiety, fear and loss of confidence. Prior expectations are important in encounters with others since they influence the arousal and flow of emotions and are ways of sustaining and changing social order (Turner and Stets, 2009:216).

Similarly, Turner (2007:179) argues that emotions represent a source of motivational energy which affects social structures and cultures. To this end, a greater understanding of social agency requires consideration of embodied agency.

Embodied Emotion and the Ontological Self

For Lyon and Barbalet (2003), emotions are embodied: *"This is because emotion, which is necessarily embodied, functions in social processes as the basis of agency. Emotion has a role in social agency as it significantly guides and prepares the organism for social action through which social relations are generated. The emotions which move the person through bodily processes must be understood as a source of agency -social actors are embodied."* (2003:50) Under these circumstances the body mediates physiological and social processes in the expression of self.

If for Lyon and Barbalet the body mediates between body and other, for the French phenomenologist, Merleau-Ponty (2001), the body provides an ontological basis for self. This is about making sense of our experiences and assessing the extent to which these phenomena are shared. This considers the social processes individuals depend on to make sense of the social world. People's perception of this begins with the body and of being in the world such that a sense of self is developed by physical action. The perception of embodied emotion does not require cognitive reflection: on the contrary, much like learning to ride a bike, we get a 'feel for it' since it is practised. This process of action, referred to as *intercorporeality*, sees that individuals act upon the world and in so doing apprehend and make sense of it (Howson, 2009:36). In this philosophy of embodiment, the feeling of this body is the connection to the world. Merleau-Ponty's ideas further ground the body as agent in social life.

81

Similarly for Scherer, (1984): *"One of the major functions of emotions consists in the constant evaluation of external and internal stimuli in terms of their relevance for the organism and the preparation of behavioral reactions which may be required as response to those stimuli."* (1984:296) This is not to suggest that emotions are merely mechanical, rather, that the complex interaction of emotion and action reflects the varying aspects of sociality, for example, integration and group formation (Collins, 1990).

Where medical sociologists such as Lyon and Barbalet (2003) focus on power in interaction, phenomenologists lack discussion of it. Similarly, the activational aspect of emotion, experience and expression and the way this connects to the body is limited. Though these emotions are mediated by social and cultural contexts, they are still driven by biological forces (Turner and Stets, 2009). These ideas compare with the more organismic and well known qualitative works of Arlie Hochschild (2003) who also drew upon the symbolic interactional approach of Goffman. It is this perspective of emotional management, which I now explore to elucidate ways in which people respond to their work with the public.

Emotional Management

For Hochschild (2003) drawing on Freud, emotion is important in signifying danger and is therefore more than a biological sense in our prior expectations. As she explains: *"Emotion, I suggest is a biologically given sense, and our most important one. Like other senses – hearing, touch, and smell – it is a means by which we know about our relation to the world, and it is therefore crucial for the survival of human beings."* (2003:229)

As with other senses, emotions are the means by which the social world is known and the way individuals relate to it. From this perspective we gain a view of emotion which is unique among the senses in that it is related to *action* and *cognition*.

From the organismic perspective of Freud, Hochschild obtains a sense of the 'signal' function of feelings and what 'gets done' to emotions from Darwin before returning to the interactional orientation by considering how social factors mediate people's expectations and the feelings they signify (Hochschild, 2003:229-230). This forms the basis for her 'emotional management' approach, where she considers the relationship between emotional experience, emotional management, feeling rules and ideology. This ideology is about the feeling rules which inform emotions and feelings. In contrast emotional management concerns the type of work involved in order to cope with the feeling rules.

Arlie Hochschild's researches concerning emotionality and expressivity are important to the discussion on emotion, since her qualitative approach to analysis considers not only the representation of these emotions but the way they are regulated by the self and others.

Following observations of the work of air hostesses and the airline industry in her research, Hochschild, employs two models in her analysis of emotions. In the first organismic dominant model in which emotions are defined, feelings are universal. Their expression is the 'surface' from which physiological changes in response to external stimuli are represented. Emotions then are the biological responses that are experienced by all and which are instinctive. These sensations for example, 'knots in the stomach' need to be acknowledged and interpreted as such, in order to derive meaning as a feeling. Further, these meanings are defined according to the social and cultural context from which they arise. This explains why Hochschild draws upon symbolic interactionism and upon the ideas of Goffman's presentation of the self in everyday life to analyse the link between the body, self and society.

From her observations of flight attendants (from recruitment to training and employment), Hochschild suggests that for the main part, their work was in helping people to relax. They did this by undertaking 'face work' such as smiling and being 'friendly', to place passengers at their ease.

Yet this type of work represented a form of emotional control over attendants which was reinforced by training processes which focused upon 'niceness' towards others such as paying customers. This acting nice and restraining one's frustration, observed Hochschild, meant attendants were continuously monitoring their emotions to ensure external expression matched what the airline company expected. This monitoring forms the basis for Hochschild's 'emotion system' which she refers to as 'feeling rules'. More widely, these rules are recognised by being self-reflexive about our feelings and the way in which others assess our emotional display, and by the sanctions which we impose upon ourselves and those which come from others. While these rules may vary from culture to culture, and from one social group to the next, these rules are taken for granted in that they set the norms by which feelings are judged appropriate to accompanying events (Hochschild, 2003:59).

Termed as 'techniques of interpersonal exchange' by Hochschild, smiles, tears or touch involve a form of acting which is performed at the surface or deep level. Surface acting implies changing external appearance or adopting pretence as a way of giving an impression of feeling. For example, in the service industry, a client may display anger at a hotel receptionist for perceived poor service experienced at dinner. Yet, the employee may be bound by the hotel company code and acceptable cultural code of response which would be to smile, nod and deal with the matter courteously. Though, this experience may feel threatening, it is handled professionally. A form of 'deep acting', refers to working on a particular feeling in order to change it and would mean the receptionist would feel 'sorry' towards a customer who was abrasive. Yet as Hochschild observed, this performing can be deleterious for some, ending as it does in burn out, depression, insomnia and eating disorders. Thus, emotion work can be seen as a 'dramaturgical distress' the consequences of which emanate from occupations which involve the manipulation of feeling in dialogic exchanges.

The point for Hochschild is that these feeling rules concerning emotion work become official culture since they are set by (mainly) male upper class superiors to suit their own disposition. Further, emotional labour occurs in employment which requires personal contact with the public, and the monitoring of this emotion work by superiors. Moreover, it is in these subordinate positions where women are traditionally found and in work which emphasises their capacity to do emotion work (air hostess, nursing etc.). In light of these interpretations about the work of emotion, it can be seen that emotions concern the interaction between the physiological, social practice and culture. Further, these techniques of emotion are not merely expression but are embodied in that they are a culturally specific technique which signals the potential or not for a specific form of interaction. Indeed, bodily gestures and facial expressivity reinforces cultural ideas concerning appropriate conduct to accompanying situations.

Similarly, for Howson (2009: 30), our bodies and our faces portray to others ideas about who we are, encouraged as we are to be 'connoisseurs of masks,' manipulating facial expressions and gestures to create impressions. Thus, the face can be seen as an aspect of the body which reveals and conceals what we are feeling. It is between emotions as embodied experiences, their social nature and relation to feelings of self and personal identity that a sociological understanding of emotions comes to light.

Having discussed more broadly the sociology of emotions, it is to fuller accounts of their relevance to the medical encounter I now turn. In so doing, I illuminate how emotions provide the missing link in the sociological understanding of these exchanges in perinatal loss encounters. In particular, the emotionality and their expressiveness by midwives and doctors are considered in relation to the training of health professionals and to the organisational structure in which they are situated.

Emotionality in Medical Training

While the study of emotions is a subject of increasing inquiry by sociologists, there remains a dearth of knowledge concerning the work of emotion in medicine. Indeed, several writers have considered the importance of professional attendance to the emotional expressivity of patients, yet analysis of such encounters is limited (Atkinson, 1995). Rather, attention is given more readily to emotion as measurable phenomena such that indices can score the quality of health and emotional well being of patients (Baker et al, 1996). While this represents a technical focus on care more generally, for Baker et al (1996) the socialisation of professionals in their training in part, explains varying emotional responses in the medical encounter.

Emotions then represent obstacles to practice since 'appearing competent' is the primary task facing students of medicine and, thus, appearing knowledgeable in front of peers. Similarly, Atkinson's (1995) research on medical education in the UK found that having the right answer equates with professionalism. Though this applies more to technical competence, it

86

can be seen that image making is synonymous with acting confidently. This performing provides a way for students to feel safe, confident and familiar with their subject. Thus, in effect, medicine is an emotion management strategy which is learnt in training (Smith and Kleinman, 1989:61). Indeed, it can be seen that the skills acquired at this critical juncture of a medical career are both academic and emotional.

Similarly, for Good (1994:65), students become active participants of the socio-cultural process by which 'medicine constructs its objects', and in so doing, develop ways of observing and speaking with others. Moreover, it is in this being with patients in the final years of training that students learn to 'write up' about others, which is critical to the understanding emotional expressivity in medical encounters. For in this writing, they learn about the subjective experiences of the patient and learn that this is time consuming.

Similarly, Thompson's (1984), concern regarding British medical encounters, hints at the irony of the situation, citing as he does about the medical interview: "*it is the one thing which distinguishes medicine from veterinary medicine. Despite being the cornerstone of medical practice, it is often seen as a tiresome interface between the doctor and the disease.*" (1984:87) What is critical here is that this distancing from patients is in direct opposition to humanistic standards of care are so publicly espoused by medical agents and educators (Baker et al, 1996:178). Moreover, the structural conditions of the working environment together with a medical subculture explain why an attempt to humanize medical training is complex.

This training socialises trainees towards skills other than listening. Where there is a story to be told, it is seen as an indulgence, and carried out when the work of medicine is completed (Baker et al, 1996). For Turner (2007:126), the social structure of the institution imposes on individuals via the micro–dynamic forces of status and roles. In playing out these authoritative positions, students then learn, and indeed seek to affirm, their status which affords them a level of power and prestige, albeit a junior one.

These roles are the conduits by which macrostructures exert pressure on encounters. Such micro level forces are the contact point between individuals and the larger scale structure of the institution. In this respect, medical professional training teaches the conditions by which to perform emotion work and with it an understanding of the hospital culture, structure and expectations.

Emotion work in medicine is more than about coping with pressurised work in an environment more concerned with presenting than talking to patients, which is an emotional strategy learnt in training. It is a learning which reflects the Cartesian bifurcation of the mind from body discussed earlier in this chapter, and which forms the basis for the practice of modern, scientific medicine in contemporary western societies. Similarly,

Turner (2009:67) argues that this separateness of mind from body, reason from emotion and biology from culture, reflects medicine's interest in an 'objective' body, compared to a 'lived' body and in part, explains its 'dis-embodied' approach towards patients. Though these perceptions are more in keeping with the largely male domain of doctors, it is within these institutions where the idea of emotion as additional work is conceived. This explains why the largely female cast of midwives is expected to perform emotion work more generally in this medical as well as social encounter.

The difficulty, however, in explaining varying professional approaches to this work lays at the juncture of divisions in practice of emotional expressivity by some though not all in the profession. It is in these differing responses to which I now turn, to suggest that where feelings are felt, they are not necessarily shown. The problem for the patient or in the case of this study, bereaved parent, is when emotion is ripped away from the situation to which it is attached.

Emotional Work in Medical Encounters with Perinatal Loss

Having considered the extent to which trainees are socialised to 'perform' in certain ways, it is useful to once again define the work of emotion in relation to the discussion on health professionals. As Brotheridge and Lee (2003) explain, emotion work is the: *"effort involved when employees regulate their emotional display to meet organizationally based expectations specific to their roles."* (2003:365) In the context of perinatal loss more specifically, it can be seen that midwives' primary task is to provide bereavement support to men and women. Yet research concerning parents' perceptions of professional responses to stillbirth and neonatal death is substantial and indisputably frames such reactions in a negative light (Sorensen and Iedema, 2009:9). Similarly, Kohner and Henley (1997:48), in writing for SANDS, found that many parents' received poor hospital care following the death of their babies.

This research is in keeping with Lovell's observations of professional practice in the early 1970s in London and her later research with bereaved mothers' in the 1990s. Lovell's (1983) reference to the ' *rugger pass'* in her findings defined the way in which babies' bodies were 'flung' about in an institutional system which sent mothers home with *'indecent haste'*. These are actions which are both insensitive, and deleterious to bereaved men and women. The dearth of policy in relation to disposal of baby's bodies and support of women mirrored that of concern for what the death of a baby represented, which was nothing more than a disappointment.

Lovell (1997:38), later associated the paucity of support with the notion of temporal collision in that the birth and death were perceived as one and the same and in effect cancelled out one another. Lovell's findings raise important questions about medical encounters in perinatal loss and the extent to which professionals are supported by their institutions in distressing situations.

Several authors (Fenwick et al, 2007; Leon, 1992) concur that health professionals receive limited emotional support and as a consequence engage in what James suggests is 'surface acting' by detaching inwardly from the distress of a patient. In part this relates to Obholzer's (2005) ideas concerning working with loss, since he argues that death represents a sense of powerlessness, the effects of which are like "emotional toxins". Similarly, Sorensen and Iedema (2009), argue that toxins (anxiety, guilt, and powerlessness) lead to professional vulnerability and in some instances 'burn out', absenteeism and even resignation.

Indeed, Gardner's (1999:128), study of midwives' experiences of perinatal death, in the UK, USA and Japan, found that a sense of helplessness was felt, such that professionals questioned their sense of worth in medicine following the death of a baby. Gardner attributed this to a lack of opportunity to acquire increased knowledge, a lack of mentored experiences and a paucity of personal and emotional support. Gardner's findings suggest that emotionality and expressivity in the medical encounter in relation to perinatal loss is hard work. In part, it explains why some professionals detach from the situation while others choose a form of deep acting and some engage in post death rituals, such as attending babies' funerals (Harvey et al, 2008). Though the latter represents the nursing sorority on the neonatal ward more generally, it compares significantly to Lovell's stillbirth experiences discussed earlier. What these studies show is that professionals can offend against Hochschild's 'feeling rule' when emotion is undermanaged or over- managed. For example, a midwife's emotiveness towards a patient's may be regarded as 'unprofessional' by colleagues (Sorensen and Iedema, 2009).

By detaching from emotional situations, professionalism is upheld. Caught between one rule and another, emotions are self-assessed and in turn assessed by others. This would suggest that if there is a micro basis of social order in the profession it stems from the arousal of emotions among individuals as they navigate encounters lodged within macrostructures.

Though these professional responses to loss vary, it can be seen that Turner's (2007:127) notion of the coherency of 'corporate units' concerning the impact of the macro-structure (institution) on the micro level of the emotional encounter, is dependent upon the coherence of the 'corporate unit' (maternity ward).

Much like Hochschild's corporate feeling rules, Turner's *corporeality* concerns the conditions by which these feeling rules are enacted. This is dependent upon clear and concise rules, where individuals have an understanding of their role and what is expected of them which represent a unified and coherent approach. By contrast, those 'corporate units' that do not have clear boundaries are ambiguously experienced. In these units midwives may be unsure when the work of emotions is to be invoked. This helps to explain why the neonatal death encounters in the literature are perceived in a more positive light. Here, some babies are expected to die for example, due to prematurity.

Therefore, ways of handling these encounters become 'visible', and practised. Thus, the micro dynamic forces of roles and statuses are manifestations of a culture of corporate units (maternity ward, neonatal unit) which are either coherent or constrain the formation of positive medical encounters. Where there is clarity then it is more likely, for Turner that expectations are met. By contrast, incoherency accompanies defensive mechanisms and emotional transmutations.

Feeling rules, together with emotion work and interpersonal exchange make up an emotional system. In so doing, they enable professionals to assess what the worth is of shedding a tear or of an inward attempt to feel sad for the bereaved in their care (deep acting). Though this displayed tear is homage and a way of paying respect to those situations where sadness is owed, it is homage to a rule about paying respect.

Feeling rules provide the basis for exchange and settling what we owe in these accounts. This is specifically linked to the findings of Gardner's, Harvey's and Lovell's research concerning neonatal death and stillbirth experiences and professional accounts of loss.

What is significant to the neonatal medical encounter is that unlike some parents experiencing earlier perinatal losses, parents and professionals on the neonatal ward have a time preceding the death during which they have dialogic exchanges and ways to relate to each other and to the child. It is in these encounters where meaning, personhood and parenthood come to be defined and acknowledged. This compares with Lovell's more negative findings concerning women's stillbirth experiences.

It can be seen in the neonatal and stillbirth findings that the expression of professional emotion differs, precisely because of the meaning attached to the event more generally. In this respect, emotion work in stillbirth experiences are poor because meaning attached to this form of loss lacks a cultural as well as a medical meaning. While this could be viewed in relation to perinatal loss more widely, the neonatal death findings from Harvey's study, (where nursing sisters engaged in memorialisation rituals, e.g. funerals, taking photos), reflect dialogic exchanges where a greater sense of emotional payment has been made. It is in these emotional accounts where a greater potential for dialogic exchange to personify the baby can occur, precisely because the baby lives longer.

From these dialogic exchanges it is possible to get a view of emotional conventions at play and how they bear upon deep acting since they apply directly to how one should feel. This provides a point of reference from which professionals can see their own actions and gestures in relation to convention. For example, attending babies' funerals is granted since it concerns institutional feeling rules about propriety of place and timing and emotional expressivity of such losses.

From Gardner's and Lovell's findings it is possible to observe what 'gets' done to emotions and how feelings are a preamble to what gets happens to them which are consequential for both parties in the medical encounter. From the organismic orientation of Freud, there is the sense of the 'signal' function of professional feeling and what 'gets done' to emotions from Darwin. These resulting occupational, hazardous emotional toxins socially interact in medical encounters since they mediate people's expectations and the feelings they signify. Thus, it can be seen why much of the criticism concerning health professionals in relation to perinatal death stem from parents' subjective perceptions, in that they vary so widely (Condon, 1986).

This understanding of the medical encounter in relation to perinatal loss is complex not least given the influence of other factors, in particular, the paternalistic nature of the medical encounter. To this end, the profession is characterised by its monopoly of a body of knowledge and specialised training which is self-regulating. Further, professionals adopt status shields to imply authority in an occupation which is fundamentally based on the separateness of the mind and body which is but object and observed. The problem in this wisdom is that our social realities are about making sense of experiences and assessing the extent to which these phenomena are shared. This emphasises the social processes individuals depend on to make sense of the social world, not the philosophical questioning of the mind and body.

Therefore, it is the experience of medicine as the dominant discourse on perinatal death which is problematic here which can be viewed in relation to a socio-political discourse more widely. This concerns policies and legislation which ascribes personhood to a human being. In the following discussion concerning foetal personhood, I argue that the medical and socio political discourse is incongruent with men and women's painful reality of the loss of their child.

Foetal Personhood

There is substantive literature concerning professional perspectives on perinatal loss. Yet there is a dearth of understanding the way in which legislation and policy shape attitudes, values and beliefs concerning such phenomena. Alongside culture, the family and other social institutions, the socio-political system is influential to a person's sense of self. This is particularly relevant to parental identity in relation to stillbirth and neonatal death. It is this which is at the core of issues about personifying stillborn children and those who die on the neonatal ward, since it relates to the way they are defined by the socio-political and legal discourse.

Traditionally, the birth of stillborn children has not been recognised, only the death by issuing a death certificate to enable the final disposal of the body (Lovell, 1983). The personification of stillborn babies became more of a socio-political issue due to a paediatrician's (Jolly, 1975a, 1975b,1976) concern with the emotional ill effects of loss due to the paucity of legal and medical certification. In relation to perinatal death, a 'Certificate of Disposal of Body' *without* the baby's name was all that had signified the presence of a human being. It wasn't until the latter part of the twentieth century that the Health Education Authority in London published a leaflet to raise awareness of the emotional impact of stillbirth within the profession. Yet these health agencies legislated upon issues of personhood without reference to the meaning of the child for parents.

Rather, legal definitions of what constitutes a person became medicalised with pathological reference to signs of life. For example, a stillborn child is defined in law as: *" a child which has issued forth from its mother after the twenty–fourth week of pregnancy and which did not at any time after being completely expelled from its mother breathe or show any other signs of life."* (Stillbirth Definition Act 1992, Schott et al, 2007:171).

94

A child who is born and later dies is defined as a neonatal death accordingly:-*"Death before the age of 28 completed days."* While seemingly arbitrary, these definitions came about to protect professionals from prosecution since they clarify when medicine is able to intervene.

As with medical discourse, the socio-political system has an integral role in the construction and deconstruction of the personhood of the baby and that of the status as a mother. As the feminist writer Linda Layne (1990) asserts, women are encouraged to view their unborn child as a precious item until they are born dead and are at a juncture when their status as a person is diminished in society. Yet the shock of stillbirth initiates a phenomenon which contradicts the fundamental premise of a women's health discourse of pregnancy and birth, and that it is a joyful experience which can be controlled (Layne, 2003:241).

Indeed, there is an abrupt end in the identity construction process; an unravelling of a woman's lived experience and a deconstruction of her motherhood. This raises important questions about defining foetal personhood according to the socio-political and medical milieu, the boundaries to which change as technology and medicine prolong the lives of those children that are born ever more prematurely.

The socio-political and medical discourse in highlighting identity is unable to acknowledge either the importance of roles played by individuals or the consequential effect of the disjuncture between biological parenthood and social parenthood.

This is reinforced by social expectations of the pregnant woman's role to be undertaken following birth. Once motherhood is assured, with stillbirth and neonatal death it becomes lost, since the identity of the child is problematic and with it, its integration into the family, community and society. The extent of this integration, it is argued, serves to affirm or deny the status of mother and father to the child in varying ways.

This is considered in light of bereavement interventions in hospital as recommended by voluntary organisations and the parental accumulation of emotional artefacts in relation to the child. As with other children, some parents acquire memories and mementoes which they attach to family narrations.

Memorialisation and Post Death Rituals

For Layne (2003), gift giving is a central social practice in establishing and maintaining a social identity and is used strategically by bereaved parents to address the problems borne of foetal personhood. Further, this gift giving can be viewed in direct relation to exchange gestures and signs of feeling with others. Moreover, the process of giving which begins during pregnancy continues through into support groups which seek to value the child and take the social credit to which members feel entitled as mothers.

Gift giving and parental construction of foetal personhood is significant in the context of stillbirth and neonatal death since the latter implies a greater number of people engaged in the process of creating an identity. Further, class, religion and spirituality act in this process and influence the way goods are used following loss. For example, in terms of class, Layne contends that members of support groups are essentially middle-class and it is this which affects the way individuals use goods and artefacts to construct personhood, as is a belief in the afterlife via religion or non-secular frames of reference.

More recently several online forums such as the www.littlefootprints.org and Gonetoosoon.org provide a number of ways in which to memorialise the person who has died. The former set up by a bereaved mother following the death of her baby is a part of what has been referred to as the 'dot. commemoration generation' which is changing the way society mourns (Greene, 2010:52). What sites such as these represent are 'Virtual Graveyard's', a place where the bereaved can 'light' a virtual candle, leave a poem or their story for others to read. That they are popular is evident with Gonetoosoon.org which to date has attracted over 3,000 visitors.

What is important about these sites is that they can be visited at any time and from a computer which may be situated in the private confines of home. That the site is visited more from midnight onwards is a testament to the nature of grief and the inevitable sleepless nights. Further, such forums are established by bereaved men and women and demonstrate a shared understanding of grief. They provide a way to pay tribute and to receive support from on-line friends.

Online forums and the accumulation of artefacts represent ways of memorialising the child who has died. Other forms of memorialising may take lace in the hospital such as taking photographs of the baby. Though the latter has been informed by voluntary organisations in response to parents negative experiences, they represent memorialisation practices none the less.

Thus, the collection of medical images and artefacts (sonogram images, photos of the baby, handprints, footprints and locks of hair) are all post death activities which serve to personify and establish the existence of the baby.

While it is tempting to view these approaches as models of good and sensitive approaches, they also imply varying practices and it is this which is important to note. For example, some hospitals employ bereavement midwives, while others don't. Similarly, some midwives encourage memorialisation in relation to bathing and tending to baby, while others refrain from these activities (Malcarida, 1999). Moreover, much of the emphasis upon good models of care comes about through bereaved parents' localised activities in fundraising and in lobbying maternity liaison committees, and it is this which prompts change in small ways. In an attempt at more standardised approaches to bereavement care, voluntary organisations (SANDS) have developed a series of guidelines (Schott et al, 2007) as recommendation for good practice in relation to perinatal loss to which I now turn briefly.

Professional Guidelines

The agenda behind more recent guidelines stems from a critique of the way health professionals respond to bereaved parents and the lack of standardised and co-ordinated systems to manage such an event (Kenyon, 2002). Traditionally, parental experiences with health professionals had been shared with the voluntary sector and viewed in a negative light such that it had emotional ramifications for men and women. For example, these concerned deleterious reference to the baby ("ugly little thing") and their meaning to men and women ('try and have another one') and a lack of encouragement to be with the baby (Kohner and Henley, 1997). Due to these experiences, principles of good practice in relation to perinatal death have been developed by SANDS.

For example, one guideline recommends that parents whose child dies in stillbirth and neonatal death are encouraged to create memories (dressing the baby, naming them and making funeral arrangements). Other principles of good practice are those which suggest facilities such as a separate bereavement suite.

While these recommendations are critical aspects to parents receiving appropriate and sensitive support following perinatal loss, the guidelines risk being subject to varying interpretations dependent as they are on the corporeality of the maternity or neonatal unit. Moreover, these guidelines are at risk of becoming 'ticklists' more in keeping with the organisational aspects of health professionals work, at the expense of providing appropriate intuitive and sensitive support. This is not to suggest that the guidelines are a futile attempt to enact change. On the contrary, men and women (via voluntary organisations) act as agents of social change, each trying to influence the political and medical agenda, albeit in small ways.

What remains is that the substantive body of knowledge pertaining to perinatal loss recognises the emotional consequences, yet fails to acknowledge some of the ways they impact upon professionals and how this permeates their approaches in the medical encounter. It is in these interactional exchanges that the relational aspects of emotion are exposed and consequential for bereaved men and women.

An awareness of the emotional consequences of perinatal loss, and ways to support men and women needs to form part of both the trainee midwifery curriculum and professional ongoing development (Layne, 2005). Indeed, much of the literature written by professionals about follow up support posits that ongoing development and awareness of loss forms a crucial part of providing sensitive bereavement care, especially that which personalises parents' experience in terms of their needs.

Conclusion

Whereas the preceding chapters have been concerned with multi disciplinary approaches to understanding experiences of death, dying and bereavement, this chapter has explored a sociological understanding of emotions. This raised philosophical and ontological questions regarding the human embodiment of emotion in relation to nature and culture and how this applied to the medical encounter. From these discussions it was shown that the emergence and development of the self and its relation to society poses a problem within sociological orientations.

Though there is a tradition within sociology on examining the self in relation to social interaction, its reference to the bifurcation of mind and body and rational and irrational emotion conceals the significance of embodied emotionality. Indeed, Lyon and Barbalet's contribution exposed the significance of the body in human emotions, particularly in relation to power in interactional exchanges. Similarly, it was to Freud, James and

99

Darwin's organismic instinctual givens and to Goffman's interactional approach that Hochschild turned, to show how facial and bodily control together with corporeal norms were critical to the presentation of a competent self. This was discussed more widely in relation to the public service industry, particularly to the training of health professionals and to the work of midwives and neo-natal nurses. In these medical encounters corporate structures and a micro and macro understanding of performing emotion work influenced professional approaches.

This corporeality suggested that professional management and control of emotions was dependent upon the coherency of the institutional unit where such encounters are situated. Consequently, emotions are not always controllable and manageable which together with micro and macro understanding of emotions in part explains varying professional approaches.

The phenomenological approach to embodiment showed how sensory experiences contribute to the ontological basis of self and in relating with others. This is despite exposure to western Cartesian influences which privileges rationality as the basis of self. I argued that this sense of objectivity in relation to emotions represented that of a medical discourse more widely yet was consequential to parental and foetal identity. This was considered in light of the socio-political aspects of perinatal death to which stillbirth and neonatal death represented a challenge. This was discussed in relation to memorialisation and post death rituals which are not informed by medical discourse but by social actors.

To this end, the experience of professional care as framed by a medical discourse reflects the contradiction referred to in previous chapters. Knowledge about death and dying has been medicalised and in the socio political arena legalised with little reference given to meaning, which in effect marginalises bereavement as a social experience.

The health professional as framed within a medical discourse lacks a corporeal coherent script and it is this which creates confusion, since they are tasked with providing both the medical and social aspects of care, yet respond in varying ways. In this context, a parental response to the death of their stillborn child and or infant is mediated by social relations in society by the social political legal aspects (which informs medical practice) and by medical discourse.

In chapter 4, the ideas of contemporary heuristic researchers such as Frank (1995) and Etherington (2004) are used to underpin empirical research which explore the narrative accounts of loss by men and women who have experienced the stillbirth or neonatal death of their child, and which build upon existing research about perinatal loss, parental bereavement and identity. In chapters 5- 8, the findings of the research undertaken are explored in-depth and an evaluation is made of using this approach.

CHAPTER 4. Research Methodology

> *"When we use our own stories, or those of others, for research, we give testimony to what we have witnessed; and that testimony creates a voice."* **(Etherington, 2000: 17)**
>
> *"The emotional force of a death derives less from an abstract brute fact than from a particular intimate relation's permanent rupture. It refers to the kinds of feelings one experiences on learning, for example, that a child run over by a car is one's own and not a stranger's. Rather than speaking of death in general, one must consider the subject's position within a field of social relations in order to grasp one's emotional experience."* **(Rosaldo, 1989:2)**

Introduction

This chapter outlines how the research concerning parents' perspectives on grief and loss following the death of their child was conducted. I begin by discussing the value of employing narrative inquiry as a methodology, given that data collection in this study comprises listening to and recording parents' narratives.

In adopting a reflexive methodology to research, I valued the autobiographical and feminist approaches of Etherington (2006:16) and Letherby (2003:7). Their ideas concerning the use of the 'self' in research include a consideration of the relationships, between the 'self' as researcher and 'others' as respondents' and the research process and product. I therefore contextualise myself in this research since this has informed the methodology within this study.

The use of my 'self' in research is not confined to discussing my researcher pathway and how I came by this topic. Rather, the 'self' is also considered in light of subjectivity, my closeness to the subject matter, the power relationship between respondents and my 'self' and dealing with emotional issues around such a sensitive subject. Further, this more reflexive consideration of research reflects where I stand in relation to my choice of design, fieldwork, and data analysis, editorship of the data and presentation of the findings.

A qualitative approach to researching grief and loss has been employed as I wished to explore parents' experiences about the death of their child and the meaning of this loss based upon their own interpretations. I was aware from other research (Leon, 2005:2; Neimeyer, 1999) of the difficulty inherent in using quantitative research methods to analyse emotional responses. Indeed, much of the research in relation to parents' experiences of loss have been conducted by medical professionals, and essentially framed in a positivist light. This approach emphasises validity and reliability and thus, 'measures' emotions as a way of explaining experience. Yet, in my discussions with parents prior to this research, I observed alternative ways in which individuals express their grief (e.g. narratives, poetry, journal entries, art work and photographs).

These are avenues of expression, I argue, in which the meaning and emotions from an aspect of one's life story can be further explored and become a way of overcoming the limitations of the spoken language. This is in keeping with other research which values narrative analysis as a valid means of knowledge generation in research (Frank, 1995; Keeling and Nielson, 2005; Josselson, 1999).

In this qualitative endeavour, I explain how I undertake narrative inquiry by utilising Mauthner and Doucet's (1998) voice relational method to analyse transcripts from interviews. I argue that while this approach is more labour intensive (requiring the reading and re-reading of transcripts), it nevertheless represents the trade-off between a long drawn out process and the richness of the data that is provided by the narratives. To this end, I adopt a qualitative and sociological approach to provide an account of responses to loss which values emotions.

Narrative Inquiry

The methodology within this research is based upon narrative inquiry and underpinned by a heuristic framework. Narrative heuristic research is a term that encompasses a large and diverse range of approaches and, thus, there is no single agreement as to what this constitutes (Mischler, 1999). For the purpose of this study a heuristic method is about collecting, analysing and re-presenting people's stories as told by them.

Heuristic frameworks assist in disentangling stories by recognising the concerns being addressed. For Frank (1995:24) these heuristic frameworks are not the truth of stories which has been the tendency of modern researchers to present their typologies. Rather, the frameworks I present from respondents narratives are a means of heightening attention to stories which are their own truth. The stories which are told may be those of wreckage and of chaos, but they are not necessarily about lives as they were lived, but as experiences of those lives (Frank, 1995).

Thus, a narrative of stillbirth and neonatal death is not confined to the death itself but becomes the *experience* of the death in this thesis. The social scientific notion of reliability and of getting the same answer to the same question repeatedly does not fit here. Life moves and so stories change with that movement and, thus, the experience changes.

In keeping both with Frank, (1995:3) and Etherington (2004:75), the narrative inquiry I employ is based on the following worldview:

- **competing narratives represent different realities not simply different perspectives on the same reality (Freeman, 1993).**
- **narratives give voice to who we are, and represent and shapes social reality (Bruner, 1991; Frank, 1995; Ochberg, 1994).**
- **the telling and re-telling of an aspect of one's life story enables a person to create a sense of self (Burr, 2009 ; Frank, 1995).**
- **re-visiting and telling one's story helps to create a sense of meaning (Bruner, 1990)**
- **we live in a storied world and lead storied lives (Howard, 1991; Mair, 1989, Sarbin, 1986).**

These approaches suggest that one's reality and knowledge is socially constructed and based upon the premise that knowledge is entrenched in historical and cultural stories, beliefs and practices (Crossley, 2000). In so doing, they challenge modern certainties since they question how we come by this knowledge. For Etherington (2004), narrative inquiry is particularly relevant since it serves to portray ways in which people experience themselves in relation to a culture. Similarly, for Josselson (2004: 2), narratives are where the memories, the representation of others, and time are all interlinked through stories into a 'fabric' that people experience – and can tell – as a life history. Thus, narratives can become the linguistic means by which the connectedness of human experience which has been lived can be expressed, and the meaning of life made explicit. Moreover, this approach provides agency since within people's stories, the self emerges.

In this thesis, where stories may differ (a couple's account of the loss of their child), they are explored for their differing realities not competing perspectives about the same reality.

Narrative inquiry has a particular value since it provides respondents with the opportunity to tell an aspect of their life story in their own words without censure. This is in keeping with Frost's (2004:7) research on pregnancy loss where women felt they were able to talk more openly about their experiences in ways which they would not usually with others. In so doing, the women were able to remain close to the depictions of their own experience and tell their story with a heightened sense of understanding and insight. It can be seen with Frost's research that the demands for the interviewer are to be with the respondent being interviewed and to understand the world from their point of view.

At the forefront of this approach is awareness that these stories are reconstructions of life events which has a bearing on how the stories are shared, which particular part of the story is told and how it is presented and interpreted. Essentially, it is the meaning of past events which change over time and which reshapes a story as it courses towards its end and which is still in process. To this end, narrative inquiry is particularly relevant in exploring experiences related to real events and which have personal meaning for the story teller who in this research, is the parent. Having discussed the value of employing narrative inquiry in this research, I set the research in context and discuss how the research came about

Context of Research Concerning Parents' Perspectives on Grief and Loss Following the Death of their Child

This research about parents' experiences of grief and loss in relation to their stillborn child or infant stems from my own personal experiences of the unanticipated outcome of a birth at forty two weeks, which resulted in the death of my daughter two days later. This experience has provided access to baby loss support groups and bereavement networks and has influenced the way in which this research has been conducted. It was imperative therefore that the data from other men and women's experiences of loss be discovered according to methodology which would reveal: "*qualitative depictions that are at the heart and depths of a person's experiences.*" (Moustakas, 1990: 38).

I wanted to be able to provide respondents with the opportunity to tell their story in both verbal and unspoken ways. This meant that entries from journals, poetry, art work and photography formed part of the narration in interviews. This affords a depth of exploration which values multiple voices, truths, perspectives and meanings. In so doing, it values individual and personal subjectivity and is recuperative for the story teller. Thus, it was with the very real sense that parents' stories needed to be heard for what they were which were representations of a lived experience which guided the purpose of the research. This did not detract however, from the need to both recognise and acknowledge my own autobiographical influence to this research.

Including the 'self' in Research

While the concept of 'self' as a major tool in the research process has been highly valued by several researchers ((Etherington, 2006; Letherby, 2003; Moustakas and Douglass, 1989; Etherington, 2006; there are many ways in which autobiography can be included in research. For example, Linda Layne (2003) in writing about miscarriage draws upon her own experiences of multiple miscarriages when she sets into context how her research came about concerning feminist accounts of pregnancy loss in America.

My own forays into previous research centred upon issues of subjectivity and clinical reliability in keeping with more positivist approaches to methodology. Yet, these were studies in which I barely mentioned my influence to the product or research process. Indeed, as Letherby (2003:142) argues, just as respondents do not tell us every detail about their experiences on a given subject; neither do we as researchers include all aspects of ourselves in writing in research.

While I have not included myself as a respondent in this thesis, reflexivity has been central to the research process. I am able to refer to the similarities and differences between my 'self' and respondents and about the way this research has led to changes in my own feelings and understanding about stillbirth and neonatal death experiences. That this is not expressed as vividly in my field work journal (yet, was much discussed in supervision) demonstrates the complexity of including the 'self' in research.

Indeed, including my auto/biographical self in the research process has been insightful and challenging since I have been caught between two conflicting notions. In my work (with bereaved men and women) I have been encouraged to be reflexive and to see my 'self' and my knowledge about the subject as a tool. Yet, in writing this thesis I have questioned the legitimacy of this approach to wider academia such that this reflexivity would be viewed as self indulgent, narcissist even, and thus, lacking in objectivity, which in more positivist approaches is highly valued.

I was reassured by the ruminations of Oakley (1992) who argues that reflexivity and autobiography are neither a form of 'navel gazing' or a means of 'self adoration'. On the contrary, 'self adoration' is much different from engaging in a critical scrutiny of the 'self' in research and thus, having insightful self awareness.

Similarly, Letherby (2003) argues that it is possible that those researchers who choose to refrain from critical self awareness in the research process could be construed as arrogant for presuming that their influence to the research product and relationships with respondents would be wholly unproblematic.

By acknowledging myself in the research here I make it explicit that I am a researcher, with multiple identities and this has influenced the research process and product.

Indeed, my initial outlook towards this research subject was one of excitement and anticipation. The former owed much to my own experience of loss which continued to be misunderstood and under-researched (from a parental perspective) and this provided a way in which to redress the balance of competing voices (professional, counselling and autobiographical literature).

My enthused approach to fieldwork was evident in that I had always favoured this particular process to research (interviewing people who generated richness to the data collected). The sense of uneasiness which followed however, concerned obtaining sufficient amount of people to conduct research with. In addition to respondents and my own sense of coping in the interview and when working with the data (i.e. transcription and analysis).

I was also concerned with bringing about a topic in which men and women may find it emotionally difficult to talk about. Having obtained these wounding narratives, would I do justice to these experiences? While these issues were at the forefront of my priorities in previous research, it was to the narrators (respondents) of stillbirth and neonatal death where I felt a particular responsibility. My sense of protectiveness towards these men and women were exposed by the use of codes I had originally attached to their names and of those of their children (both deceased and living) to their accounts. Yet, by later attaching pseudonyms throughout narratives, accounts of loss were easier to follow throughout the thesis and were much more personal.

This did not detract from the ethical obligations of this research (i.e. anonymity and consent). On the contrary, the sensitive subject made the need for ethical procedures much more explicit.

Ethical Procedures and Gaining Access to Respondents

This research involved contacting men and women whose children had died as a result of stillbirth and neonatal death. The fact that this was a subject that resonates closely to my own experiences meant I felt obligated to consider my motives and ability to engage in this research not only for myself but also for respondents. That these men and women mentioned that one of my identities as a bereaved mother was helpful for them was reassuring.

Ethical approval was sought from the University of Bristol Ethics Committee prior to contacting voluntary organisations to elicit support in recruiting parents whose children had died. As with any study conducted by UK tertiary educational institutions, sociological research is subject to ethical review (Lee, 1993:28). Since there would be no recruitment via the National Health Service or Government institution, or any organisation which received government funds, there was no requirement to seek ethical approval from any UK Local Research and Ethics Committee (LREC). Previous experience as a researcher had elicited significant insight into the processes and the time required to obtain approval from LRECs. It was therefore decided that there was insufficient time within the context of this particular research to be able to obtain ethical clearance according to these means.

Due to the sensitive and personal nature of the research I was conducting, access was sought via my membership of the Stillbirth and Neonatal Death Society, SANDS, whose aim is to support bereaved parents. SANDS have been established for twenty-five years and is a resource for parents and health professionals. With a network of approximately two hundred support groups across the UK and a Helpline, SANDS aim to provide a way for men and women to talk about their experiences of grief and loss in confidence.

Accessing respondents through support groups was a critical starting point at which to invite parents to participate in the research. Indeed, I was aware from other research that obtaining respondents becomes more difficult, the greater the sensitivity about the subject under investigation (Lee, 1993:60). Accordingly, SANDS and other organizations (the Birth Trauma Association and babyloss.com) were approached to access potential respondents. The Birth Trauma Association and babyloss.com permitted access by posting a notice of invitation to the research on the chat room which parents used on their website.

SANDS provided six support group facilitators to contact. Following initial phone contact or a meeting with a group facilitator, copies of the introductory letter (Appendix A), research information sheet (Appendix B), Consent Form (Appendix C) and contact details were provided for respondents who required further information. The information given to respondents outlined that they were under no obligation to participate and could withdraw at any time (Newell, 1993:113). Further, the data collected was to be treated in the strictest confidence.

While a printed name and signature were asked for on part of the consent form, this did not detract from the need to seek verbal and ongoing consent throughout the interview process (Lee, 1993: 103). Of the six support group contacts provided, I met and spoke with three facilitators who distributed information about the research to support group members. This was repeated with a further group facilitator who submitted information to the support group committee for review and approval prior to distribution. SANDS were approached once again but declined a request for other group contacts. While the reason for this was not supplied, their suggestion that information about the research could be posted on their website was taken up.

To obtain more respondents I attended the SANDS annual conference and annual general meeting in October 2006. It was evident from the presentations SANDS delivered that their focus as an organisation was shifting towards increasing and formalising their research activities. Traditionally, SANDS' role as an organisation was to provide a location in which parents could share their accounts of loss by telephone, support group or through the World Wide Web chat room. Yet with the temporary cessation of the chat room (which was popular), many of these voices would remain unheard.

This was because SANDS had to close the chat room following negative exchanges between bereaved parents concerning the death of a child following a medically advised termination. Despite this, the SANDS annual conference provided contact with two women who agreed to participate in this research.

Through another support group facilitator I had met previously, I was able to successfully recruit (6) men and (21) women. This created a 'snowball' method of research. As one parent was interviewed, so other parents who had spoken to those who had taken part in this research became interested in being interviewed. Parents would leave their contact details (with other parents who had been interviewed) so that I could contact them. While this method was successful, this sample comprised of men and women who were articulate and self-reflexive and who were able to voice their experiences. While I was committed to encapsulating the experiences of both men and women from varying backgrounds and despite, other sources of recruitment already listed (World Wide Web), membership of groups comprised mainly of women.

As with the cessation of the chat room, other unexpected issues impacted upon the research process. My original intention was to recruit men and women whose child had died following a 38 week (full-term) gestation.

Yet, despite these original 'respondent characteristics', men and women were talking about experiences which varied not only in terms of gestation but how they came about. While I saw this as a possible limitation and how this may affect the product of the research, unlike a large scale, government funded project, I welcomed the flexibility afforded my position as sole and principal researcher and was able to respond and be encouraged by these varying experiences which only added to the richness of data.

For example, a feticide narrative (Chapter 5) represented a critical narrative which remains publicly silenced yet, which reveals much insight as to the complexity of an experience concerning the death of a baby.

I was aware of the difficulty from other research (Frost, 2004; Letherby, 2003) in encapsulating the experiences of both men and women which are insightful. Indeed, while there were articulate and self reflexive men willing to be interviewed there were clearly those who were not. Letherby (2003) suggests that the difficulties in recruiting men in research about the loss of a baby may be gender specific in that they maybe too embarrassed to talk to a female researcher about the topic.

The limitations to recruitment were not confined to men, but to younger women who have experienced the death of their child. For example, younger respondents may have provided accounts where they were expected to cope as they had their whole lives ahead of them compared to 'older' women in this thesis who were expected to cope by having a replacement child. Similarly, the perspectives of men and women's children may have illuminated respondent's experiences further, though this has ethical implications. For example, in order to investigate children's perspectives, I would have needed to conduct more ethical procedures with the UK police force and with each County Council where I was investigating.

Given the highly sensitive nature of the subject being researched, my concern was therefore to ensure the protection of the respondents which I was able to recruit. For example, the initial introduction with parents by email or on the telephone enabled me to outline the research and to address any concerns they may have such as length of interview and any issues of confidentiality.

This way of communicating enabled me to gain consent, to send information and learn about a deceased child's birthday and death anniversary thereby initiating an interview at other times whilst acknowledging that any day may prove distressing for respondents.

While the majority of men and women approached provided consent, two women withdrew their consent and declined to be interviewed. These women were at the earlier stages of a subsequent pregnancy and were anxious around the time of ultrasound scanning appointments. Together with recruitment and taking note of important days for respondents, subsequent pregnancies show the practical difficulties involved in conducting this highly sensitive piece of research. However, this informed the amount of information respondents were sent including details about the research and consent.

Telephone contact initiated consent to send information to potential respondents which comprised an introductory letter (Appendix A), research information sheet with my telephone contact details (Appendix B) and consent form (Appendix C). The information sent out to potential participants provided contact details, the aims, objectives and purpose of the research and why one-to-one interviews were being sought.

Contact sheets (Appendix D) provided contact details and help line numbers for support organizations such as CRUSE and SANDS. For reasons of safety and sense of security, respondents were provided with the opportunity to be interviewed at a venue that was convenient for them (Franklin, 1997: 84).

For example, at their place of work, in their own home or at a relative's home. Some women felt better able to take part, if interviews took place in their own homes because they knew that relatives or husbands would be present in other parts of the property.

Other respondents had young children and were interviewed at home. Part of the reason for recruiting respondents through support groups was to ensure my own safety. In keeping with other research (Craig et al, 2002), I undertook procedures (informed others of the interview, start and end times) which would facilitate this. Having described the means by which respondents were recruited, I now turn to describe the characteristic details of the sample of men and women in this study.

Details of the Sample

Between October 2006 and June 2007, six men and twenty-one women were recruited to participate in interviews across the UK. Of the twenty-seven respondents who have been interviewed, their age ranges are indicated in Table 2.

Table 2. Frequency of the Chronological Age of Research Respondents

Age	30-34	35–39	40-44	45 +	Total
Frequency	8	8	10	1	27

Of the twenty-seven men and women who participated in interviews, one respondent, a father who is fifty-two years of age is placed in the forty-five years and above frequency. This is necessary given the significant difference in chronological age of this respondent to the rest of the sample which raises a very important point. While not of the same family, there are two respondents who are forty one and fifty-two years of age respectively, yet each experienced the death of their baby thirteen years ago.

Thus, the age of the sample is not an indication of the age at which respondents experienced the death of their baby. Rather, as the over thirty years of age variable age range suggests, men and women have different lived experiences of loss.

Another possible explanation as to why respondents who are aged thirty years and over agreed to be interviewed, is that as members of support groups (at one time or another) they may have had the opportunity to rehearse their story (since they have told it several times) and are therefore more confident and used to talking about their experiences.

The aim of the research was to obtain narrative accounts of loss from both women and men. Apart from one father, the men comprised of the partners or husbands of the women who had been interviewed.

Each parent who represented a couple was interviewed separately at different times, often on different days and in some cases, in different locations from one another. As more women than men have taken part in this research, it could be argued that the disparity by gender is because men are more reluctant to talk about their experiences. Yet this does not seem to apply to the men interviewed in this research given that men's narrative accounts of loss were similar if not greater in length that the women's. Further, these men were able to express their grief as openly as the women (e.g. by crying) when telling their story. A further explanation may be found in the fact that while the men attended a support group at some stage (usually soon after the death of their baby), unlike the women, they did not all continue to attend these groups. Only two men took part in predominantly female occupied groups which meant opportunities to recruit men were diminished.

Recruitment to the study was open to any member of the UK population who as a mother or father had experienced the death of a baby, and indeed interviews took place in the North and South of England and in large urban centres and in town and rural locations. There was no interest forthcoming from men and women from ethnic minorities through the World Wide Web or support group.

It could be argued that membership to support groups was mainly representative of white British men and women. Yet this cannot be corroborated as the identities of support group members remain confidential by the guardianship of support group facilitators who act as the gatekeepers to guarantee members protection. As such, these findings cannot be generalised to mothers and fathers from ethnic backgrounds or a younger or older cohort of men and women who have experienced loss.

Of the men and women who were recruited, twenty one were married whilst the remainder were with partners (n=4). Two participants were divorced and were single.

Table 3. Frequency of Research Respondents Employment by Occupation.

Occupation	Frequency
Education	4
Health care	6
Civil service	1
Computing	1
Retail	3
Voluntary work	4
House person	4
Study	3
Other	1
Total	27

The majority of parents (n= 18) were employed and occupied variable and diverse positions in teaching at primary, secondary and tertiary level. Other respondents were employed in retail as shop assistants. Of those respondents employed in health care services these comprised reception work, nursing, managerial and physiotherapy. While seven males and four women were engaged in fulltime work, other women (n=8) had undertaken part time work. The 'other' category represents a respondent in banking at managerial level. Interestingly, the other eight participants who were women described themselves as occupying a variety of roles with four being house persons, four engaged in voluntary work with SANDS and three engaged in part and full time studies. While part-time work and being a house person suggests that women may be taking a career break to look after their young families, each mother described how, prior to the death of their baby they were ambitious and once occupied successful and 'high flying' positions. Yet following the death, these women felt unable to resume the same job as fund managers, nurses and engineers. Instead they worked as shop assistants for a few hours, became volunteer fundraisers and house people.

Other women changed career following the death of their baby and were studying for first degrees and PhDs, the subjects of which were perinatal loss. A further observation of respondents' occupation is that the sentiments of colleagues in response to loss deterred some men and women from returning to work.

The location of a baby's death varied yet was important in mediating parents' responses to loss. For example, some received empathic support, while other respondents did not. This is informed by the current literature and the findings in Part Three about respondents' experiences with health professionals. Of the fourteen respondents whose babies were stillborn, seven took place in local hospitals while a further seven babies died in large city or teaching hospitals. Their gestational ages at death are presented by Table 4:

Table 4. Frequency of Stillbirth by Gestational Age at Death in Weeks

Gestational age at death	Frequency
20-24 weeks	3
25-29 weeks	1
30-34 weeks	0
35-39 weeks	6
40 -44 weeks	3
Total	13

The gestational age of death of stillborn babies ranged between twenty three and forty four weeks, with the latter being four weeks past the respondent's estimated due date (upon the recommendation of professionals). Altogether, thirteen respondents experienced a stillbirth. Though these deaths represented a tragedy for respondents, for some the deaths were unexpected. For others (n=7) they were expected since it had previously been identified that the baby had died in the womb, and this had been detected by women (not feeling any movements) and ultrasound screening. This compares to the experiences of men and women whose baby lived for a brief time.

Table 5. Frequency of Age of Neonatal Death in Days

Gestational age at death	Frequency
Under 1 day	7
1-5 days	3
5 - 10 days	0
10 - 15 days	4
Total	14

Of the fourteen neonatal deaths, ten took place in large city hospitals, since this is where the technology and specialist professionals (neonatologists) were located.

For example, one baby was born in a local hospital and transferred to a London hospital for specific treatment. The hours that babies survived ranged between two and seventeen hours, and between two and four days respectively. Four respondents spent between twelve and fourteen days with their baby although this was at times confined to touch through an incubator. These experiences compare with respondents stillbirth encounters with health professionals.

Men and women's neonatal ward experiences describe nursing staff as empathic interlocutors. The neonatal death experiences also provided relatives and friends the opportunity to meet the baby and to acknowledge their existence to respondents' social network. Further, siblings could visit and, thus, be a witness to the baby's place within the family history. Twelve participants had young children (under the age of five) when their baby died.

The impact of other losses such as miscarriage was explored by four women in this study. These represented 'early' miscarriages between six and eight weeks respectively. Multiple miscarriages during twin pregnancies also took place for one respondent at ten, twelve, and fifteen weeks respectively. The majority of respondents had another child following the death of their baby as indicated in Table 6.

Table 6. Frequency of Subsequent Children Born

Subsequent Children	0	1	2	3	Total
Frequency	1	8	11	7	27

While one respondent had not had a subsequent child when interviewed, she was experiencing a subsequent pregnancy at twenty-four weeks gestation. Though these figures represent surviving children, the deceased baby continues to form part of respondent's familial history.

For example, photographs of the baby adorn respondents living rooms and in some cases bedrooms and in so doing represent the baby's place within the family. The baby is both remembered and commemorated for many years. This is irrespective of the number of years which have lapsed since the death as indicated by Table 7.

Table 7. Frequency of Time in Years Since the Death of the Baby

Time in Years	Frequency
Under 1	2
1-4 Years	11
5-9 Years	7
10-15 Years	6
Total	27

Of the twenty-seven respondents, two women had experienced the death of their babies three months prior to the interview. Though these represented recent deaths, I did not want to exclude parents from having the opportunity to tell their stories. I was appreciative of the sentiments of a facilitator (gatekeeper) who agreed it was important that parents had the choice of whether or not to approach me. Several respondents (n=11) experienced the death of their baby three years previously, which, as Rando (1991) argues, can signify a time when parents may experience a worsening of symptoms of grief.

While this is not an easily identifiable trend in these parents narratives, the expectations by friends and family that a parent should no longer 'dwell' in their grief, is. Yet parents' narratives suggest that a death which occurred three months ago compared to a death ten or fifteen years previously, evokes a response which reveals intense sadness. As Rando (1991) suggests, parents reflect upon the death of their child as though it happened yesterday.

Indeed, the years which pass since the death comprises a series of significant events that can serve to compound parents sense of loss and grief. The birthday, the first day at nursery, to their last day at school before making their way in the world, all mark a transition into childhood and adulthood of which the parents are denied the experience of.

Having described the characteristic details of the sample of men and women of this study, I now discuss how the research was conducted.

Conducting the Research

Prior to interviews, four focus groups were conducted with parents to guide the themes of the research schedule in addition to what I wanted to ask in interviews. Respondents who expressed an interest in attending the focus group at the initial telephone meeting were sent a letter of invitation (Appendix G), and upon completion a letter of thanks (Appendix I). Focus groups took place in participants' homes to provide a sense of agency and comfort, and away from any clinical setting (a hospital environment) where it may have caused distress (where the child had died). One of the focus groups comprised of a 'women only' group and the second group comprised of a 'men only' group as it related to themes specific to motherhood and fatherhood. Permission from respondents to tape the groups was granted and assurance was given that all of the comments would be anonymous and treated with confidentiality and upheld as per the ESRC (2007) guidelines. Respondents who were unable to attend the groups were invited to write comments on the themes the particular group was focusing upon.

In recognition of the sensitivity of the subject matter, between four and six respondents took part in each group. Referred to as mini focus groups, Krueger and Casey (2000), contend that such groups offer distinct advantages in that they provide a greater opportunity for all members of the group to speak and fully express their views. Similarly, focus group respondents in this research demonstrated a whole range of emotional responses to the experience of grief and loss which informed the research schedule (Appendix F). Given the highly emotive subject matter, I discussed what motivated respondents to take part in this research.

Respondents' motivations

Respondents' motivations for participating in the research ranged from wanting to help my 'self' as the researcher while others felt they wanted to 'raise awareness' and 'educate people'. Those wanting to assist the research stated that their 'voice would be heard' and that 'people need to understand this' (impact of the death of a baby).

It was at this juncture that it became evident that while my motivations were similar to respondent's (raising awareness) they also differed in that I had 'intellectual privilege' over that of respondents. This is not to suggest I had superiority. Rather, I had the resources and materials available to transcribe and disseminate experiences which many respondents did not. This does not suggest either that respondents are unable to represent themselves, on the contrary some do so willingly (lobbying parliament see Chapter 8). Rather, it was to my 'self' as the researcher who respondents turned to make their anonymous voices more 'public'.

It was for this reason that interviews provided the basis by which to engage reflexively and consider notions of power and the work of researching such sensitive issues. This reaffirmed the sense of ethical and moral obligation that this subject demanded during interviews.

The Interview Guide and the Interview Process

> *"Narratives show how fragile our existence is and how quickly such well- being can be destroyed."* (Layne, 2003: 177)

In addition to focus groups, interviews were informed by literature on narrative analysis, researching sensitive topics and parents' published narratives (Etherington, 2006; Kohner and Thomas, 1995; Lee, 1993). A pilot interview with two women further provided the means by which to expand the interview guide to include those issues which previously had been omitted. Pilot interviews provided a way of attending to any unanswered questions, particularly those which are sensitive and to be approached after rapport and trust had become more established (Lee, 1993: 78).

Twenty-seven respondents were interviewed (six men and twenty one women) and the research schedule (Appendix F), its purpose a guide, was by no means exclusive or exhaustive.

Following Burck's (2005:240) recommendations, this qualitative research rejected a structured format style of asking questions in a particular order to avoid repetition (the questions may have already been answered earlier in the interview). In light of recording highly sensitive and emotive narratives it was essential for stories to unfold and that the interview guide reflected this by being an open format. Thus, questions (e.g. age, occupation, and previous pregnancies) which were potentially offensive were not asked in a linear format during interviews but where appropriate or within the story as it were being told.

Several authors (Dingwall, 1997; Gubrium, and Holstein, 1998; Silverman, 1993) write about the importance of reflexive approaches to research interviewing since it is regarded as a social encounter. I was reminded by each interview with respondents how I needed to locate myself as the researcher.

Respondents were aware I was a parent of a child who had died as they had asked how I came to conduct this research. Several respondents affirmed that this part of my own story legitimated talk about an issue which they felt they were otherwise discouraged from talking about, especially among some family members and friends.

Despite the relative easiness in wanting to talk about an experience, some accounts were more private than others and with more reference to the emotional as opposed to the physical aspects of the experience. For example, I was reminded of the strength of emotion which accompanies grief and to feelings of anger, sadness, and despair. All of these emotions and more had visited me during my own experience of loss. This focused my attention on how such feelings are intimately related to ideas of motherhood and the physical reality of parenting a dead child, which for respondents in this research, remains a private endeavour. These processes (interviewing, transcribing) meant I was also faced with the question of how I reconcile myself with the various roles and positions I occupied as a researcher, parent and data analyst.

As a reflexive researcher, Behar (1996) suggests observing these differing roles and positions not as separate beings but as entities which are intertwined, albeit in a complex way. In the context of this research, this meant being prepared to expose biases, and held assumptions and in this research, my emotional responses in the collection of data. Thus, while there were opportunities to talk (briefly) this facilitated a period of self reflection which was recorded in my field journal yet, discussed more widely in supervision and counselling sessions.

This came to be a way of writing and voicing the concerns I had. For example, in one interview I had felt uncomfortable due to the negative reference by a respondent towards my own previous source of emotional support (support group). I left feeling disappointed and bewildered by someone who I thought would 'know better'.

This interview exposed the ongoing negotiation of my status as an 'insider' and 'outsider' in the research process. While the former meant my approach was appreciated for being less voyeuristic (since my interest was genuine and personal), my 'outsider' status as a researcher from an academic background meant I had to experience the discomfort of the perspective that was provided as part of the interview. I had to contend that this comprised not only the complexity inherent in research but an understanding of loss according to one's own personal values, perceptions and beliefs. Further, it was evident that while personal experience of the subject matter could in most instances facilitate rapport and enable connections, the previous experience meant that disclosing one's own interest in the research is not always desirable. Moreover, what this interview showed is that while the subject matter is an issue that the researcher and respondent may both have a connection with, it does not follow that the researcher identifies with the respondent's sentiments or perspectives.

For Letherby (2003:14) finding a balance in research is critical not least since is not always evident who holds the power. I was reminded of the tension in this power relationship from this interview and of the work of emotion in distilling one's sense of discomfort such that, Hochschild's emotional management thesis (see chapter 3) resonated deeply. It was to Lee et al (1999:6) I turned, since they assert that a personal experience such as bereavement is emotionally charged and that research

This can be viewed in light of reflexive ethnographies where the researcher begins a study based upon their own experiences. As Etherington (2006) explains: *"Our personal history, when it is known to us and processed in ways that allow us to remain in contact emotionally and bodily with others whose stories remind us of our own, can enrich our role as researcher. Our 'empathic resonance' allows us to hear the others' experiences without the need to defend ourselves against that knowing."* (2006:180)

Etherington's reference to 'empathic resonance' follows from a way of being with respondents' as well as with the 'self'. For Ellis and Berger's (2003): *"the researcher often feels a reciprocal desire to disclose, given the intimacy of the details being shared by the interviewee"* (2003:162). While I disclosed my own personal reason for this research when asked, compared to the interview described earlier, other interview encounters evoked intensely sad emotions within my 'self'. I felt much moved and had the utmost respect for such profound stories and to the men and women who shared them. Yet, unlike the more private moments with transcripts in a single occupied office, I felt I could not fully express the impact of these interviews until I attended therapeutic sessions with a counsellor as a means of coping with these processes.

Drawing on Fontana and Frey (2000): *"interviewers must necessarily be creative, forget 'how to' rules and adapt themselves to the ever- changing situations they face."* (2000: 657) Indeed, I was reminded that no two research situations are the same. Further, that both respondent and researcher are affected by this encounter. Indeed I have earlier stressed why I felt the need to 'check in' with respondents in the days following the interview, and ask them how they were and how they felt the interview went. This sense of responsibility did not end on leaving the field. It continued to influence the transcription and analytical processes in this research.

Transcribing Interviews

"One of our most difficult duties as human beings is to listen to the voices of those who suffer. These voices bespeak conditions of embodiment that most of us would rather forget our own vulnerability to. Listening is hard, but it is also a fundamental moral act; to realize the best potential in postmodern times requires an ethics of listening. The moment of witness in the story crystallizes a mutuality of need, when each is for the other." (Frank, 1995: 25)

While often used in qualitative research, the process of taping interviews and transcribing them is rarely acknowledged in the writing up of the research itself (Lapadat and Lindsay, 1999). For Kvale (1996:167), self-transcribing narratives enables the researcher to be close to the narrator's meanings. Without such explicit knowledge the reader is impoverished in their position to interpret or indeed understand the data.

Respondents were offered the opportunity to read the narratives to censor anything they felt they did not want to be included (e.g. issues of anonymity related to the naming of medical staff involved in the births and deaths of their children and on-going legal cases) and to verify that the meanings had remained intact. While the majority of respondents declined to view their narratives, three received their transcripts as a way of memorialising their child and to keep with their other 'baby items'. For others there was concern that their account of loss was incoherent. It was at this juncture that I also took further note of my 'intellectual privileges' as a researcher in terms of editorship. Indeed, several authors (Cotterill, 1992; Letherby, 2003; Stacey, 1991) contend that the researcher has ultimate control over the data since they choose which words are utilised and which can be taken away.

The dilemma within this research was not with 'doing away' with words but in keeping them. My concern was being able to include all of respondent's experiences and 'voices'. Yet, the generous level of data meant this was not possible.

While one of the original aims of the research was to present multiple voices, interviews varied in duration and, thus, some respondents had more to say than others. This has meant that some respondents appear more than others in some chapters or a particular chapter. Thus, my approach to the presentation of data was in keeping with other authors (Layne, 2003; Letherby, 2003) and which represents 'fragmented representations' of respondents' lives. As discussed in Chapters 5 – 8, I describe how I select extracts from narrative accounts of loss to exemplify groups of respondent's views on issues which relate to emerging themes. I also provide accounts which are in common with another while emphasising those that differ and receive much less attention in the literature.

My concern with representing experience also influenced my decision to avoid 'cleaning up' original text. My interest was not with 'polished' or grammatically correct accounts but with all of the *'erms'*, *'ums' and 'ye know?'* and *'it were like'* of respondent's regional accents which formed a part of their everyday conversation. To delete such words would feel like deleting an aspect of a lived experience. Further, repeated exposure to these words was an essential part of being immersed in heuristic research, since the details added depth to the quality of the narratives. As Etherington asserts: *"we are rarely aware how much of the English language is made up of incomplete sentences and incorrect use of grammar or language generally"* (2004:80). Within the narratives, this 'incorrectness' provides a clue and proffers a sense of meaning behind a particular aspect of a story.

In keeping with Etherington: *"transcripts are social constructions; they are the re-telling and re-creations of stories that have already happened and not a faithful copy of a static world."* (2004:80). Similarly, several researchers (Blum and Mc Hugh, 1984; Garfinkel, 1967) contend that narration is a complicated social process and a form of social action that embodies the link between narrator and culture.

In light of this claim it can be seen that parents responses to loss as well as their stories and how they are told are culturally shaped, a notion I explored in chapters 1-3 of this thesis. In relation to this, narratives are vital to the study of social phenomena since they are a focus on the embodiment of specific life stories.

As Josselson and Lieblich (1993) explain: *"life stories themselves embody what we need to study: the relation between this instance and that social action (this particular life story) and the social world the narrator shares with others; the ways in which culture marks, shapes and or constrains this narrative; and the ways in which this narrator makes use of cultural resources and struggles with cultural constraints."* (1993:20) Indeed, by analysing specific narratives, greater knowledge about how cultural discourse both provide and constrain resources for articulating experiences is revealed.

In summary, the purpose of listening to someone's story and analysing their narration is to explore and understand the subjective world in which the respondent lives. The interview, and the story which emanates from within it, provide a rare glimpse and therefore a rich opportunity to shed light on the psychological and social realities of the respondent's life. Further, in giving voice to parents as respondents in this way, there is an ethical and moral obligation to ensure that a narrative is not reconstructed or indeed marginalised.

This was further considered in light of Langer's (1991:168), criticisms of other writers' interpretations of sensitive interviews. For example, in writing about Holocaust testimonies, Langer argued that there was a tendency of writers such as Gilbert (1985:828), in coping with such testimonies to devise 'softening' language which diminished the severity of the impact of these experiences. Further, that the traditional historical narrative which is reflected upon in such testimonies overemphasises the 'good ending' of a story such as being liberated from the death camps.

As Langer (1991) explains from one of the interviews about prisoner experiences of the death camps in World War II: 'When American tanks liberated Ebensee (concentration camp) Sol R. (respondent), says that that he and his friend Sam, whom he had been together with from the beginning clung to each other not for joy, but because "now really the truth is going to have to come out. Up until then, it was all speculation that our parents [had] not survived, or my sisters or brothers, or anybody. Now the day of reckoning was coming and it was very frightening…. So as much as we were happy once that we were getting freed … the fact is that we go to go home to find out."(1991:169) Indeed, they found that their families had perished and this fact alone altered the relationship to the reality they tried to convey in the interviews.

Where there was hope now there was very little way in which writers such as Gilbert (1985) could make consolatory use of despite their attempts to do so.

Langer's criticisms are useful in that they reveal the instability of particular words and how they could be used or misused to support various researcher perceptions and deceptions. This does not suggest that the testimonies I refer to are comparable to those of the respondents in this study, on the contrary, such experiences need to be viewed in their own light.

I refer to Langer, since it is precisely because such testimonies can be misinterpreted that it was important to pay attention to and engage with the transcription data in this thesis. Thus, I was able to detail the emotional response of the parent as narrator. For example, by noting the expression of tears as an explanation for a silent pause (Frost, 2004: 173). Moreover, by being reflexive I commit to learn from the content of the stories and how that knowledge was created during the analysis. To this end, I valued the approach of Mauthner and Doucet (1998) who following Brown and Gilligan (1992), analyse narratives using a voice relational method.

132

Data Analysis

As with the interviews, I transcribed the focus group data and coded it on a case by case basis, to ensure anonymity and that the personal details of respondents remained separate from the data itself. By assuring anonymity, the identities of respondents remained confidential and protected as required by the Data Protection Act, 1989 (Lee, 1993:171). Following Boulton and Hammersley (1996:295), interviews were digitally recorded and promptly transcribed to ensure data was not lost, and that parents perspectives continued to inform the ongoing data collection process. Due to the large amount of data which twenty seven interviews and four focus groups generated, software packages such as Computer-Assisted Qualitative Data Analysis (CAQDAS), Atlas.ti and NVIVO were reviewed.

In consideration of these computer packages, I appreciated that software had the capacity to assist in indexing and generating separate files as well as coding which can change as themes emerge from the data.

In recognition of these objective means of analysis, there was the practical reality that narratives were subjective and could be read in so many ways. The data has been analysed by reading and re-reading the narratives several times to capture themes as they emerge (Frost, 2004: 162). The data generated by the narratives was rich and full and needed to be viewed according to both their uniqueness and similarities. I was not comfortable with the thought that I would need to somehow dilute subjectivity (respondents and my own).

In keeping with Etherington's (2004:212), reflexive model to research, I wanted to appreciate the 'messiness', depth and texture of a life which has been experienced and spoken. In so doing, it allowed for the subjectivity of the parents accounts of grief and loss and of my own subjectivity within the analysis. In this reflexive model, it was possible to move beyond any premise that this research could only be read in one way (Mauthner and Doucet, 1998:122).

This is why I valued the approach of Mauthner and Doucet (1998:125), who propose the notion of 'relational ontology' in which the individual is embedded in a complex web of intimate and larger social relations (See also, Riches and Dawson, 1997:53-75). This means that respondents' narratives in this research are explored in relation to the people around them and to the broader social, structural and cultural context in which they live (Mauthner and Doucet, 1998:126).

Following from the work of Brown and Gilligan (1992) on *Women's Psychology and Girls Development Project* at the Harvard Graduate School of Education, Mauthner and Doucet, (1998:125) describe how they analysed their own data about the experiences of motherhood and post natal depression and sister relationships within a sociological framework. This method emanates from clinical and literary approaches (Brown and Gilligan, 1992), interpretive and hermeneutic disciplines and relational theory (Brown and Gilligan, 1992).

Following from their extensive research in psychology and education, Brown and Gilligan's method emphasises the notion of relational ontology. While this idea has been theorised in political theory, feminist philosophy and feminist legal theory (Minow and Shanley, 1996; Ruddick, 1989; Tronto, 1995), Brown and Gilligan's perspective is based upon a view of humans as embedded in a complex web of intimate and larger social relations. This contrasts with previously held assumptions about individuals within liberal political thought of being rational and separate beings. Thus, relational ontology considers the self in relation to others and thus, as a 'relational being' (Ruddick, 1989:211).

This can be viewed in light of Giddens (1984), sociological consideration of individuals within their social contexts and of the interplay of social structures on human agency. The focus in this thesis then is not upon a view of humans as independent individuals and autonomous beings.

Rather, what are at the core of the analysis in this research about men and women's experiences of loss is the issue of ontological interdependence *and* both dependence and independence.

This follows the approaches of other researchers (Rogers, 1994; Tolman, 1992; Way, 1994) at Harvard University. While the environment in which these academics work influence the way they adopt and adapt such frameworks, in the context of the research on parents' accounts of grief and loss here, discussion follows about the way in which the voice relational method has been *interpreted* for use in this thesis.

In keeping with Mauthner and Doucet (1998:126), the voice relational method framework represents an attempt to transfer relational ontology into the methodology and to data analysis by considering respondents' narratives in light of the relationships to people and to the broader, social, structural and cultural contexts within which they live.

By adopting this interdisciplinary sociological approach to develop an understanding of the experience of self, some of the ways respondents attempt to give meaning to and contextualise their experience is elucidated. In this 'voice centred' approach to research, a transcript is read four times whilst listening to the original tapes. As the readings are explored so the different voices of a complex web of interactions with the world are heard and represented.

The readings comprise of four stages in this research and are outlined as follows:

1)   **Reading for the plot and our overall responses to the narrative**

This comprises two phases in which the first is to read for the overall plot of the story provided by the respondent, and the second, for the researcher to read where they are situated in relation to the story being told so that any theoretical assumptions are explored and examined. In reading for the plot the researcher is required to write about their own responses to the narrative and how they relate to the story both intellectually and emotionally. In this way, I viewed the story being told against that of my own background of experiences such as the age at which a baby died and how I responded to the parent's narrative in terms of any prompts I used, especially where my own feelings did not necessarily resonate with that of the parent's experience.

For example, my line of questioning and prompts varied according to the level and type of support respondents received in hospital.

2)   **Reading for the voice of the 'I'**

The second reading represents listening to how respondents feel and speak about themselves. In paying attention to the use of the pronoun 'I', the researcher stays close to the multi-layered voices and perspectives of the respondent. In listening and reading for the 'I', the contradictions and the times when parents experience difficulty with their emotion become apparent. Particular attention is given to the pauses and the gaps in speech as people try to articulate how they feel, and to the moments when people become upset. For example, when people describe the death of their baby or the moments leading up to when their baby died, it was commonplace for participants to stop, pause and become tearful. In taking note of the contradictions, I observed how the women in particular tried to make sense of the death and to find meaning by changing employment.

Conversely, where there were no words, the men often drew upon metaphors to describe how they felt. For example, one participant drew upon the plot of a film to define how he felt and coped since the death of his son, since the actor in the film was tasked with having to cope with emotions which were challenging.

3) Reading for the relationships

The third reading comprises listening to the way in which respondents talk about their interpersonal relationships, be it with their partners, their relatives (in particular their parents), their children, and the broader social network within which they live. This form of reading is particularly useful for exploring any perceived grief differences among men and women in the research. Further, the extent to which the personhood of the baby and the parents were validated were seen in light of the relationships with others (health professionals, friends and work colleagues

4) Placing people within cultural contexts and social structures

Respondents experiences of grief and loss in this reading are placed within the broader social, political, cultural and structural contexts. Focus is centred upon the structural and ideological factors which serve to enable or constrain a parents way of living and thinking. In this sense how individuals draw upon discourses in society and how this impacts upon parents is considered and the roles they undertook within those structures (e.g. the meaning of mother or father and parenting). This reading enables an exploration of the mother and father's changed sense of self and identity as a parent, spouse, friend and co-worker following the death of their child.

In keeping with Mauthner and Doucet's (1998:135) approach, it was only after the four readings that the data was 'broken down' into summaries and themes based on the four categories generated by the readings. This has proved useful since the data have remained intensively rich with the connections between the stories becoming clearer.

Thus, the thoughts of the parent in relation to their loss and the discourses which shape their beliefs and view of the world appear much more evident.

Conclusion

This chapter has outlined how I have conducted the research pertaining to parents' perspectives of grief and loss following the death of their child. In so doing, it outlined a narrative approach to researching parents' accounts which was viewed in light of the sensitive and emotive subject matter. This turned to the discussion on the use of my 'self' in this study and how this has influenced both the research process and product. In so doing, I have provided a methodological account of this study which describes in detail the challenges presented.

A critical consideration of this research process I have argued is an essential aspect of conducting sociological research. It provides accountable knowledge in which the details of my reasoning process have led to the findings. This formed the basis by which to emphasise the ethical and moral obligation inherent in conducting fieldwork with men and women who have experienced the death of their children and of the means of data collection.

I described how I gained access to respondents by employing a 'snowball method' to recruitment, which was the only viable way of obtaining recruits. Indeed, it could be seen that much of the reliance upon voluntary organisations and 'gatekeepers' in the form of support group facilitators meant that the results were not able to generalise experiences to other bereaved parents in the UK. Yet it was argued that the richness of the data to which a narrative inquiry afforded, provided accounts with much insight into a lived experience.

This chapter further considered the difficulties of researching a subject that exists primarily in the private realm of family life with no language or public discourse of its own. This raised questions about some of the ways in which to explore socially invisible phenomena and to bring out silent voices. This meant that the entire research process was guided by the subject matter and thus, employed a reflexive model as a way of conducting interviews and transcribing data. I outlined how this informed the means of analysis for which I valued the sociological approach adopted by Mauthner and Doucet (1998). In this voice relational method, experiences could be viewed in light of the broader social, structural and cultural world in which respondents live.

The merits of employing this approach were outlined, in particular the themes which could emerge in relation to these broader constructs and be viewed in relation to the influence of relationships with others. To this end, parents' narratives have been systematically analysed using a labour intensive approach which involved reading and re-reading and also listening to narratives several times. The tension between such a lengthy process and means of analysing data was viewed as an essential trade-off between time and the accumulation of very rich data.

Following the discussion of the methods employed in this research, the demographic profile of respondents was outlined. Particular attention was given to the number of years which have lapsed following the death of a child to emphasise the impact of such experiences as being long lasting.

These accounts of grief and loss are explored in relation to the analytical methods described in this chapter and also in relation to the theories and research outlined in Chapters 1 to 3. The following analysis chapters (5-8) draw on a reflexive approach to present data collected from twenty-seven men and women in an exploratory qualitative study.

CHAPTER 5. Reading for the Plot Within Narratives

> "I will tell you not what you want to hear but what I know to be true because I have lived it. This truth will trouble you, but in the end you cannot be free without it, because you know it already; your body knows it already." (Frank, 1995: 63)

Introduction

While the methodology chapter discussed the ways in which the interviews were conducted, this chapter outlines the overarching themes to emerge from the interviews and which are further explored in the proceeding chapters. Following discussions regarding reflexivity as outlined in the methods section of the thesis, this chapter further explores the dynamics of the relationship between the researcher and the parent being researched in relation to notions of (heuristic) research methods. This chapter then considers the ways in which both men and women contextualise their experiences of grief and loss in relation to their previous expectations about pregnancy and biomedicine alongside their perceptions of the death of their child. It is suggested that these narrative accounts can be read in relation to both the ongoing consequences emanating from the death to the meaning of the loss of a child. Before turning to the narratives, I explain what it is to read for the plot in this chapter.

In reading for the plot, the narratives are considered as constituting the social reality of the narrator. This is in keeping with other reflexive researchers (Etherington, 2004:81; Frank, 1995: 24) where the narrative is viewed as the experience and the *what* of the story and the discourse is the *plot* and how that knowledge was created. Thus, the death of a child is not just a topic of the narrative, it is the condition by which respondent's tell their story through a wounded voice. These embodied stories are both personal and social in that they are told to someone. Yet the way in which they are told is shaped by internalised experiences with others and from popular culture. It is a storytelling which differs to respondent's everyday interactions because it is private, both formal and informal occurring as it does in the present, yet preserved for the future.

It will be shown by these narratives that the plot to people's stories represents the *taken for granted* plot about pregnancy, birth and biomedicine more widely. I argue that the transition to parenthood is an essentially given and unquestionable rite, yet as these stories demonstrate, challenge modernist representations of pregnancy and birth, leading to the development of a 'no guarantees' plot within respondents biographies.

While this permeates throughout the forthcoming narratives, these stories are varying in so much as the central plot is the child yet; the sub plots are about the deaths of children who die in utero (in the womb, during pregnancy), during labour, at birth, as a result of feticide, prematurity and neonatal death. While there has been prior warning for example, going into premature labour and of a fatal risk in some instances, for others, there is no prior knowledge of an impending death. Though such death experiences vary, these sub-plots have been selected since they represent for all respondents a biographical disruption and a grief which is deeply felt over the life course. It is this which forms part of the 'no guarantee' plot when compared to the socially available plot of healthy outcomes and live births.

These popular images (smiling pregnant mums) set in place the narratives of the stories about how birth is told in popular culture and are most powerful when they reinforce habits of thought acquired elsewhere. This can be viewed alongside notions of progress and interventions in obstetrics and neonatology to which the death of a child, in particular a baby, represents a challenge to modern ideas of progress.

A case is made that these plots and sub-plots are about a death and a loss of predictability which are endemic to late modern times and to which the self stories which proliferate in respondents' narratives, are one response to uncertainty. The chapter concludes by suggesting that reading for the plot provides a way of untangling the relationships which comprise psychic life.

141

Reading for the Plot

The first reading of respondents narratives was about getting a sense of what was the overall plot, for example, what has happened, and to follow the unravelling of events and to listen to the who, what, where or why of the story which frame the subplots. I attended to recurring words, images, metaphors, emotional resonances and inconsistencies, in addition to shifts in the narrative position (first, second and third person). In this, I located the respondent and contextualised the overall narrative in relation to their situation, in terms of their relationship, reproduction, and their perception about the medical care and bereavement support they have received.

The themes presented within are not exhaustive, yet they constitute essential component parts of the plot which also appear as subplots, under sub-headings. The next section is therefore concerned with the central plot being the death of a child and the subplot of a narrative which is the experience and how knowledge around this was created. A case is made that ideas about biomedicine and its ability to save and prolong lives generates a taken for granted plot about pregnancy and birth which are endemic to western societies. It is this which ultimately reflects a loss of predictability when a child dies in the modern age.

The narratives which follow in this reading are presented as either stillborn or neonatal death and with pseudonyms to protect the identity of respondents and of those they discuss. For this purpose I record the respondent by the gestational age of the baby when they died at birth in the stillbirth narratives, and the gestational age of the baby and how long the baby lived in the neonatal death narratives.

Parental and Biomedical Expectations and Limitations

The backdrop to the following sub-plots reveals modern expectations about biomedicine, technology and advancements in public health such that death of a baby is viewed as a mistimed experience. Further, these experiences show that life saving technology has little relevance to the social consequences of the death of a child for both parents and professionals. In selecting a subplot as a demonstration of these similarities, it is important to note that respondent's were not asked specifically about their perspectives of biomedicine, rather it was a theme which was raised by respondents and later returned to as they continued to narrate their story. An example of this concerns a father whose second son was born (forty weeks) experiencing difficulties breathing, and who lived for fourteen days. In this account, the birth of his first son who also experienced oxygen deprivation at birth, yet with the intervention of medical technology survived is discussed. As the interview continues, the reconstruction of the birth and subsequent days reflects the father's grasping for an understanding about why medical technology saved his first son Freddie, yet could not sustain the life of his second child, also a boy, Ollie:

R: The labour was alright right up until the moment he was born. There was nothing to say that there was anything wrong. When Freddie was born they rushed him over to the resus trolley straight away .....[pause]. But when they brought him back there was that great sense of calm that comes over you. So when they put Ollie over to the resus table I wasn't too concerned because I remember with Freddie that was alright. But then seconds turned to minutes and then time ticked on. I don't know why it sticks in my mind but you know on the resus table I looked at the clock and at 15 minutes they still had him over there. I think that's when I realised that something had gone wrong. Angela [respondent's wife] kept saying all the time where's my baby, where's my baby. By this time there were quite a few people in the room......
Andy, father of baby boy Ollie (born at forty weeks, lived for twelve days).

This previous account demonstrates some of the ways in which medical technology shapes perceptions of surviving complicated births. It can be seen that this taken for granted plot is also shaped largely by media reportage about advancements in reproductive and neonatal technologies.

For example, Linda Layne (2003), refers to a cover printed by Life magazine in which the caption title: "*Miracles of Birth: The Blessings of Medical Revolution, Healthy Babies Who 10 Years Ago Would Never Have Been Born*", represents the taken for granted plot that babies inevitably survive. It is argued that this faith in the ability of medicine to fix the potential for a devastating outcome is firmly rooted in our cultural and social psyche. Similarly, Guillemin and Holmstrom (1986) proffer the notion that the preservation and extension of the population's life expectancy is paramount to medical progress and the belief that it can only improve is evident in the field of obstetrics and neonatal technology. Yet the expectations of a healthy outcome far outweigh that of medicine's ability to guarantee a healthy and live baby at birth.

For example, in the last decade the rate of stillbirth in the population increased, before returning to its current level (5.3 deaths per 1000 births), which indicates limited medical progression in this field more recently. The point to stress here is that despite modern achievements in life expectancy generally, the death of children on the neonatal wards, in utero or at birth remains largely hidden, which makes it a difficult phenomenon to grasp. Modern times therefore confront the individual with a complex understanding of the world and of life as it should be. This can be viewed in relation to the experience of the death in the previous narrative where Ollie's deteriorating state is perceived as a mistimed event leading to a gap between what is understood and what is expected (healthy birth as with the first son) to that of the eventual reality of the death.

Set against an emerging sense of disbelief, the Andy begins to question medicine's ability to save his son, which is evident in the paradoxical stanzas which challenge the meaning of that gap. In the second account, the father once again reflects upon his own observations of events and those of the consultant who was tending to his son in the Special Care Baby Unit (SCBU), and who he perceived was reluctant to give him bad news:

144

R: I went to see him in SCBU with all the lines and I asked if he would make a recovery. The Consultant Paediatrician said: 'yeah, yeah' he can make a recovery. He didn't give too much of an impression that there was anything too badly wrong. As time went on over the next few days we knew he was poorly and we asked if he would make a full recovery. The Consultant kept saying: 'I can't tell'. I said theoretically can a baby this poorly make a recovery, he said in theory yes, but I think he knew right from the start how bad it was but he didn't want to tell us there and then so he waited until he was absolutely certain himself before he told us the bad news……

Andy, father of baby boy Ollie (born at forty weeks, lived for twelve days).

In the second account, Andy is aware of his Ollie's deteriorating health, a fact he perceives is not acknowledged by the consultant. To ascertain understanding of this, the father suggests that the consultant is biding his time, as though waiting for the right moment. It is the sense of disbelief which forms part of the plot (experience of grief), the central part of which is the death of a child. This sense of confusion and grief continues in this narration to form a further subplot in the search for a cause of death for which there was no previous indication and which can be viewed in relation to previous expectations.

This taken for granted plot extends to the notion that advanced clinical skills and improvements in medical diagnostics can indicate the cause of death (post mortems), which more importantly provides a reason and meaning. Yet sixty percent of perinatal post mortems are inconclusive, which has consequences for parents years after the event (SANDS, 2009). For example, respondents narratives concerning inconclusive results led to continuous self-interrogation and self-blame with the majority stating: *"what if I had done this or that."* The following third account given again by Andy and demonstrates the unrelenting questioning that emanates through some of the narratives and which emphasises the brutal fact that there are no answers:

R: Since then we have been trying to get to the bottom of what happened and why did it happen? I've looked at loads of stuff on the internet. When I originally asked the consultant he said there was a lack of oxygen to his brain. Well how did it happen? It happened around the time of his birth and they couldn't place it. He gave us the impression it could have happened before the labour, well how? His explanation was that his chord could have been crushed or kinked. Enough to stop the blood going through or when the head is going down and it can get crushed like that. How long would it have to be crushed for? ....The chord blood test showed he had been oxygenating alright which is a mystery so how did he get asphyxia?.....The consultant – if there is anything that is not clear cut he won't discuss them unless we ask and that umbilical test is one of those. I looked at the internet how they do the test? They didn't keep the placenta – I had to keep asking them where it was and they admitted in the end that they'd thrown it. It might have provided answers because when it comes back that they don't know why it happened then Angela turns it in on herself and starts to blame herself even though people tell her it isn't, she still does......But we live in the twenty first century and we've got all this technology to make it safer....

Andy, father of baby boy Ollie (born at forty weeks, lived for twelve days).

Within the narrative, the gap lies between the expectation that the father will get an answer and the reality that he doesn't and never will. When there is a lack of explanation as to why the father's son died, the respondent tries to find out this information on the World Wide Web. There is a sense of unfairness which shifts from the fact of the baby's death about which nothing can now be done, to the perception of medicine and failure to prolong life to the exclusion of the baby from any definitive medical category, since there is no cause of death or explanation.

The father is exasperated, frustrated and worn out; he has nothing to turn to by which to explain and make sense of the death of his son. Similarly, this subplot is similar to the narratives given by the majority of respondents where there is no known cause of death. Yet these answers are critical since they are an attempt to understand and locate the death within existing knowledge about the world. Of note is that the narrator of this story talks about the former predictability of which there is now none.

Together, these sub-narratives provided by the father concerning the death of his son demonstrate the complex way in which the sense of meaning is constructed in relation to expectations of fatherhood and biomedicine which constitute the overall plot. The father's expectation in the first account given about medicine being able to fix anything, is not spoken of in isolation but contextualised in relation to the birth of his first son, Freddie. The seeming certainty that all will be well is shattered and replaced by a lack of control over the outcome (death of his second son, Ollie). This account is representative of the way in which expectations and biomedicine as themes, developed throughout the course of several in-depth interviews, rather than as issues which are considered and then discussed as a deliberate course of narrative. It can be seen within the previous sub-plot, that biomedicine asserts its own 'master' narrative which goes beyond the hospital and to the strategies that more powerful interest groups use to shape the culture of death.

Similarly, Frank (1995) suggests that this master narrative relates to the viability of the modern medical project which was assumed to mitigate the fear of dying by breaking down the threat of mortality through prolonging life with technology. In this context, maternity and neonatal units are but a speciality and sub-speciality designed to deconstruct this threat of death. Behind the hospital then lies the modern expectation that for every suffering there is a remedy. Yet the consequences of this biomedical master narrative is complex, not least since it requires the restitution of the bereaved back to their functioning self which in itself requires a solution of which there is none. It is as the biographies reflect; only the restoration of the child who has died can alter this fact and it is this absence of a solution which is shocking.

In keeping with respondents' narratives, those within this chapter are selected because they contain explicit examples of some of the ways men and women attempt to make sense of and find meaning from their experiences in relation to their expectations about parenthood and medicine. Thus, the links between the death and what is expected are context bound and are more implicit within certain 'subplots' which will now be explored.

The subplots concern:
- Feelings of guilt and self-blame
- Feticide in relation to self-blame
- Subsequent pregnancies and births

This is not an exhaustive thematic list, but serves to examine some of the ways in which parents accounts of their experiences of the death of their children are contextualised within the interviews.

Guilt and Self-Blame

In reading for the overall plot, the experience of the death of a child was considered central to respondents' narratives. From within these stories emerge subplots of experiences which while similar in outcome (the death of a child), vary in terms of how they came about (prematurity, death in utero, death during birth or soon after, neonatal death, and expected and unexpected death). Feelings of guilt and self-blame emerged as a recurrent and strong theme from narratives, despite these varying themes.

For Worden (2003: 125), feelings of guilt are common in any death yet for parents who experience the stillbirth or neonatal death of their baby, the '*what if*' and '*if only*' within narratives, suggest that in particular, women respondents feel culpable for the death of their children. This was a recurring and strong theme to which the women returned to throughout their narration and as the following two accounts of self-blame demonstrate.

The first example concerns a mother who experienced the stillbirth of her son. In this account, feelings of blame and guilt are discussed in relation to the choices she made about birthing her baby. Despite the reassurance given by the obstetrician who helped to deliver the baby (that a caesarean might not have led to a different outcome), what remains is a question of doubt:

R: Because he was a breech delivery it meant they brought in a sort of expert in breech delivery. He offered us the choice of um, going for Caesarean or continuing or both but things were still fine. There didn't seem any reason to go for Caesarean. Because of all the precautions he was monitored all the way through so there was no or any kind of distress, there was nothing to indicate that there was anything wrong. My only question was should I have had a Caesarean and um he said we can't explain why he died. It didn't stop me from beating myself up about it over the years, thinking what if, what if?
Wynnie, mother of baby boy Bryn (stillborn at forty weeks).

R: It was what was called an exemplary pregnancy no signs of anything being wrong. I know I have gone back over things and looked at what might have indicated that something was wrong but you know, you can ask yourself questions about what you ate and what you drank and what you did and torture yourself which I did a lot after Christopher died [baby who died].
Mary, mother of baby boy Christopher (born at forty-one weeks, lived for four days).

While the guilt felt by the mothers of baby Bryn and baby Christopher appears irrational to the observer, self-blame in relation to the death of a child is about reality testing for researchers Dent and Stewart, (2004: 173). What they mean by this is that the question (to one self or another): *"what could I have done to prevent this?"* is repeated continuously until the final reassurance is accepted that under the circumstances a parent did all they could.

Yet this differs from the findings of this thesis irrespective of the number of years which have passed since the death of a child. Respondents, in particular women, continue to self-blame as though they were able to control external events and failed to intervene.

The following account demonstrates self questioning in relation to feelings of guilt and self-blame following the death of twin girls:

R: The hardest thing was that they were alive and trying to breathe but nothing could be done to help them. Was there anything we could have insisted upon that could have been done? Everyone we asked said there's nothing they could do, but you never stop asking. Possibly my uterus couldn't cope. You always have that feeling of guilt what could I have done that never goes away even though every one tries to reassure you. That was a pretty bad Christmas to say the least........
Ruth, mother of twin baby girls Melody and Joy (born at twenty-seven weeks, lived for two hours).

In the previous narrative feelings of guilt and self-blame are formulated by questioning the self. In so doing, the respondent challenges her body's ability to bear children (uterus couldn't cope) and to nurture (breathing but nothing could be done), in this chaotic telling. This account represents a form of chaos, given that it is part of a story when listened to and is told in haste and with speed. The narrator of this story implies a lack of control over events which is complemented by medicine's inability to alter the course of events in intervening to help her daughters aspirate. It is this chaos which reveals that no one is in control, not the respondent and not medicine. The significance of this is such that it has served to undermine the respondent's knowledge and expectations about life and in so doing, has diminished her confidence in her ability to bear children.

In this unravelling story there is a sense of being swept along life's mistimed path, there is the fact of the death of her daughters and of a mistimed social celebration, Christmas. Yet the ultimate worst of the narrative are the deaths which remain central to the plot of her story.

The central challenge of this story is to listen to and to hear the feelings which the narrator has difficulty in revealing. In listening to the transcription this is evident in the hurried telling. It is at these times, when the suffering in the words can become difficult to capture unless emphasis is given to take note of facial expression and emotional expressivity in interviews. This was important in light of Frank's observations of chaos narratives.

Where this account pointed to the lack of control over events, which is a For Frank (1995), this form of narrative is one of the most embodied, for if the story is told on the end of a: *"wound, then it is also revealed on the edges of speech."* (1995:101) By this he means that such narrative is at times beyond speech, and in a sense is lacking, yet it is this gap which reveals chaos in the silence of the speech, and it is for this reason that other forms of feeling are captured in the telling of the story.

theme similar to other experiences described in this thesis, the following sub-plot to a story presents an altogether different perspective. It concerns a respondent who was faced with the very tragic task, at six months' gestation, of undergoing a medically advised termination of her baby, who had an abnormality which would result in his imminent death during birth and of a potentially harmful risk to the mother. It is a narrative which has been selected to show that while the sub-plots to stories differ, the grief and the experience of the death of a baby is a loss deeply felt by all men and women in this research.

Feticide in Hospital

It has previously been argued that the death of a child, in particular a baby, is difficult to comprehend not least because it is relatively hidden from the social networks to which we relate. Yet feticide is considered socially and culturally incomprehensible since it describes doctors terminating the life of the child in the uterus (by injecting analgesia into the baby's heart) in hospital.

Several authors (Statham, 2002; Zeanah, 1989) posit that parents whose babies died as a result of feticide experience an intensity of grief as would parents of babies who are born spontaneously. Yet parents who face the difficult decision to end their baby's life due to a life threatening health condition, are not only likely to feel extremely anxious and distressed but also experience a profound sense of guilt, shame, doubt, failure, and loneliness (Schott et al, 2007: 116).

While termination can be medically recommended, other authors (Ashurst and Hall, 1989:116; Hunter, 1994) argue that it can mean women feel as though they are killing a part of the self. The additional burden of ending the pregnancy in some instances can lead to severe trauma and post traumatic stress disorder (Kersting et al, 2005).

In the following account, the narrator talks about the tragic circumstances surrounding the death of her son at twenty-four weeks gestation and who was diagnosed with hydrocephalus (the severity of the baby's condition was such that the baby's brain would be protruding from its head if he was born following nine months gestation). The narrator and her husband had been informed by a paediatric neurosurgeon that a preventive operation had never been performed in which the baby survived. The mother, Holly had to wait two days between the feticide and the induction for the birth, which occurred twenty four hours later:

R: The picture was so bleak and I can remember being in complete shock obviously and being numb and believing it wasn't happening. I feel awful about it all [upset]...I can't stop crying every time I tell it. It was very traumatic. I can't believe they're making me do any of this, making me inject something into the baby's heart and then wait with a dead baby inside me then go to hospital to be induced. We were waiting for two hours in the waiting room knowing what was going to happen. I kept going up to the desk and said you know we are here to see somebody and we're booked in, we're not just here for a scan they know why were coming. She just said oh well we're way behind. We went into the room and people started scanning me again. My husband got pretty angry as you can imagine and said what are you doing? They said aren't you here for a scan? They had no idea why we were there. It was just awful....This was my first pregnancy I had no idea what I was dealing with. We had no support at all and I just remember going through the whole day crying and thinking how am I going to get through this. I just want to get in my car and drive away, I don't think I can go through anything else. I had decided that somehow I had killed, murdered my baby and I was very anxious how I would be looked at and judged..............

Holly, mother of baby boy Ben (stillborn at twenty-four weeks).

In the previous account, the mother makes an explicit connection from the way her baby died to feelings of guilt and self-blame in this account of her story. There is a sense of loneliness and helplessness in a situation worsened by the care she received. Of note is the fear of being judged which can be seen in relation to self-blame, since this has been strongly identified in instances where people see their misfortunes as a result of their own actions. Similarly Archer (1999:141) suggests that self-blame and judgement stems from the belief that people generally get what they deserve. While a rather harsh and inhumane notion, it nevertheless helps to explain why the mother of baby Ben felt intense self-blame following the feticide of her son and expected to be judged.

The previous account has been selected not least because the centrality of the plot is once again the death of a baby. The protagonists and the parts which make up the story about why the death occurred is important, since the experience of grief, while similar to other accounts is nevertheless in terms of loss through feticide, even more complex than much of the literature and professional accounts of loss suggest.

153

Given this dearth of knowledge, discussion about the feticide narrative is speculative. It can be seen that this account, the most prominent feature of which is being judged, represents an essentially moral stance more widely in society on two counts. In the first instance, this can be viewed in light of Foucault's discussions about medical regulation of people's bodies and behaviour, which I discussed in Chapter 3 in this thesis. To this end, this fear of being judged relates to medicine's regulatory stance on the nation's health and of providing 'safe guidelines' by which individuals are expected to adhere, in particular pregnant women.

The point here is that pregnancy has its own rules of social behaviour that women are expected to follow (good nutrition, no smoking or alcohol) and as a consequence, pregnancy becomes a public experience, a bump to be touched and shared with the rest of the world. Similarly Howson (2009:129), in writing about the body and society, argues that expectant women are scrutinised both professionally (antenatal screening, ultrasound scans) and more widely in the community by friends, colleagues and the media. It is this obstetric gaze from hospital to the community which opens women's lives to scrutiny and, it is argued, to guilt and to feelings of self-blame which have been expressed throughout women's narratives in this thesis. It is this fear of not having done something right (eating, drinking and so on), during the pregnancy which stands out so prominently in these accounts, none more so than in the feticide narrative where the fear of being judged occurs precisely because it is expected.

This understanding of pregnancy and bodily experience as shaped by a medical and political discourse reinforces this sense of a fragmented and alienated self which is presented within the narratives. It is argued that the second reason for expecting judgement in the feticide narrative concerns a moral discourse within the political arena.

Until the last decade or so of the twentieth century, the Abortion Act 1967, (in relation to all cases of gestation) was subject to significant political and social controversy and it is this which is considered with the feticide narrative. Despite its benefits in reducing maternal mortality, between 1969 and 1971 there were eight attempts to reform the Act by Conservative party politicians'(Simms,1971). While the medical profession were initially divided as to its benefits, by 1980 over fifty organisations allied to medicine, social work, the women's movement and trade unions were in favour of the Act (Simms, 1981).

While it is not within the remit of this thesis to discuss abortion in relation to perinatal death more widely it is, nevertheless an important feature of the feticide narrative and one which provides a way of explaining the respondent's fear of being judged on a much wider social, moral and political level. Just as women are subject to the obstetric and public gaze during pregnancy, similarly the unborn child has become an object of obstetric scrutiny and as a socio-legal subject worthy of ethical debate and moral discourse. Described by the medical fraternity as a foetus, the unborn child's emerging identity in the latter part of the twentieth century in medical terms at least has been notoriously challenging, the parameters of which have been widely discussed in Chapter 3.

The personification of the baby is important to respondents in particular in terms of their place in the family. For both men and women in this research there was a very real sense of frustration which permeated through their narratives in relation to having subsequent children.

This frustration was borne of the assumption by others that another child could act as a replacement for the baby who died, and, thus, liberate respondents from their grief. A case is made that this contrasts with respondents' accounts, the majority of whom experience intense anxiety and terror during the pregnancy, the labour and birth.

Subsequent Pregnancies and Births

It is widely reported by researchers (Dent and Stewart, 2004; Schott et al, 2007; Wallerstedt et al, 2003) that a pregnancy following stillbirth or neonatal death is one of overwhelming anxiety and mental anguish. Despite these effects, support during a subsequent pregnancy in respondents' experiences is varying. In part, this could be explained by professional interpretation of an article by Cain and Cain (1964) concerning 'replacement child' syndrome. While dated, they suggest that a child born following the death of another somehow replaces the pain of the loss of the child who died. This has been challenged by Grout and Romanoff's (2000) study of bereaved parents who had subsequent children following the death of a baby. Their findings suggest that it is not the child which is replaced; it is the space that is created by the loss. While this may represent a physical space per se, the accounts given by respondents about their experiences in this thesis, suggest that they continue to experience an emotional void despite the birth of subsequent live children. This represents the grief and the loss of the child who died which is felt continuously over several respondents' life courses:

R: It doesn't matter how many babies we do or don't have you can't ever replace the baby you lost. There is always something missing, my family isn't complete, it's never going to be complete because she is not here. It's how you feel.... a complete and utter emptiness and that is how I felt after I had Lucy [baby who died]. That hole has been left here now, there is a permanent gap there where there is a whole part of my life that should have been................
Isobel, mother of baby girl Lucy (stillborn at forty-two weeks)

R: I don't want this baby growing up feeling that we only had her to replace them and if we could go on to have another one or ten babies and if time and finances allowed us we would......
Sophia, mother of baby girl Elen (born at twenty-four weeks, lived for two hours).

R: There is this idea that if you have another one somehow it makes it all OK you know, but it actually... I've had two children and I would have liked to have shared my life with Beth [baby who died].
Paula, mother of baby girl Beth (born at forty weeks, lived for seventeen hours).

156

These narratives demonstrate that the child who died is irreplaceable since they are firmly entrenched as a part of the mother's sense of self, her biography and family history. What varies between these respondents is the number of subsequent pregnancies they have experienced resulting in a live birth. As their words imply, their experiences of birth, death and subsequent pregnancies and birth once again differ, yet what remains in each narrative is the emotional void and pain of the loss of the child who died. It is this which represents the ultimate challenge to respondents more widely in the community particularly when meeting with others socially: -

R: I met with a friend of Mum and Dad's and she said I'm really sorry to hear what happened. Then it was: *"are you are going to have another one?"* Even if we do have another one it will never replace Samuel [baby who died]. People think because it s a baby you didn't know him or her you can just have another one and that'll be fine.........
Briony, mother of baby boy Samuel (stillborn at forty-three weeks)

These accounts suggest that the replacement child discourse proffered by Cain and Cain (1964) has extended from hospital to the community more widely, evidence of which can be found in the previous narrative.

It can be seen that other people's responses to the death of a baby such as that by the family friend owes much to a sense of personal vulnerability at being exposed to their own familial mortality. This is an issue which is supported empirically by other researchers. For example, Snyder (1997) found in her research concerning graduate students' perceptions of mortality that respondents overestimated their age of potential death despite reference to actuarial tables about average ages of dying and causes of death. While this may reflect the attitudes of a young generation who see their whole lives ahead of them, this more reassuring outlook is not shared by the respondents within this thesis. Rather, there is the very real sense of mortality which owes as much to the death of a child who is overall central to the plot, and to the potential loss of further children. It is this which invokes the anguish and the fear of so many subsequent pregnancies, some of which are demonstrated as follows:

157

R: If I have a problem and if I can't got hold of someone [midwife] and by the time I can I'm hysterical because it took me four hours to get hold of someone .If I could get hold of someone in the first five minutes all I would need is for someone to reassure me and I'd be OK. I don't think people realise how hard it is cos you feel quite guilty really that you are having another one.......
Sophia, mother of baby girl Elen (born at twenty-four weeks, lived for two hours).

R: It was incredibly stressful, subsequent pregnancies are incredibly stressful. And the birth, I was incredibly worried about that. I felt it was important that I should be treated differently and I should be able to ask for things if I needed to. Yeah, I thought that was really important, that I was treated differently. Because it's not the same after you have lost your baby, pregnancy will never be the same again....
Wynnie, mother of baby boy, Bryn (stillborn at forty weeks).

The previous narratives have been selected since they represent for the majority of women in this research a distressing experience. Both accounts provide evidence of distress and terror. This contrasts more widely with the literature about pregnancy and birth and less upon ways to support women following loss.

Other than the more recent perinatal loss guidelines written by Schott et al (2007), there is a dearth of literature concerning ways to support both men and women through subsequent pregnancies. Indeed, the following account demonstrates that men suffer as much anxiety as women in this study:

R: Wynnie [partner] was incredibly keen to get pregnant as soon as possible and I wasn't at all. For me it just seemed like the last thing I wanted to do at that particular moment in time. The idea of doing it having had that experience was like Oh my God you must be insane! You want to go back to having that experience again you know what I mean? Even though everything rationally said it would be fine, that wasn't even the point.... The point was for me that pregnancy and whatever could happen afterwards was just so utterly terrifying...But Wynnie was in just a desperate state that I kind of saw that was the only way forward for her, so I felt like I kind of what's the word?......................

I kind of sacrificed my own instincts in that situation and you know obviously looking back it was entirely the right thing to do. You know my instincts on this occasion were in some ways entirely wrong. Well not wrong just different........

Karl, father of baby boy, Bryn (stillborn at forty weeks).

This account demonstrates that fathers as well as mothers have fears. The narrative also reveals the anxiety about the lack of guarantees. This relates to the taken for granted plot and to the wider contradiction in medicine and in feminist writings. For example, where feminists (De Beavoir, 1972), have attempted to unmask medicine as an agent of social control with reference to the way women are treated and defined as weak.

By comparison, men's biology is viewed as running an even course without crises and, thus, defined as strong. Implicit in this are medical definitions which frame reproductive disorders in women, yet invisible in men. As Rillstone and Hutchinson (2001), point out, women may seek out the construction of medical categories as ways of finding meaning to their embodied experiences that represent disruption to their lives for example finding the causes of death, and questioning their reproductive ability. In so doing, are they not active participants in the construction of discourses that define their embodied experiences? What of men's? Including men as well as women in this way of thinking about pregnancy in relation to perinatal death changes such debate, since what is implicit in both men and women's narratives is the significance of the taken for granted plot about pregnancy and reproduction itself.

Indeed, for the respondent in the previous account, his reproductive capacity as a man is not guaranteed neither is his status as a father, until his second child is born and when he feels like he has become a father for the first time with the birth of his second child:

R: Obviously it's different for the father. They have no, very little physical relationship to that baby, to that body, whereas for a mother they've had a very intimate experience with that body. I was focused on – Wow we've got a live baby, you know and being properly feeling like a Dad for the first time. In that sense I didn't feel like I was when Bryn [first son] died even though in some ways I did. To me it didn't feel like I was a father. Wynnie very much felt like a mother I think after Bryn died. Maybe it's a gender thing, maybe it's just an individual thing, I just don't know…For me, I was kind of like no we haven't got a baby therefore I am not a Dad. The way that I related to Bryn was like he was a man already, you know the way I described how he held us. He didn't feel like a baby in a lot of ways, he felt like somebody I knew intimately and someone who I have spent a lot of time with strangely……
Karl, father of baby boy, Bryn (stillborn at forty weeks).

The previous narrative defines the juncture at which he becomes a father. A different relationship is formed with his deceased son and continues now as though he is a grown man who holds his father in his deepest moments of grief. This respondent's journey to fatherhood however is mistimed and, hence, fearfully anticipated throughout the subsequent pregnancy of his partner. Moreover, it is explicit in its account of the effects of the taken for granted plot surrounding pregnancies and birth and ideas concerning fatherhood.

Indeed, there was a sense of ambivalence which prevailed throughout men's narratives which while also experienced by women in this research, differed in its intensity. The struggle which respondents describe extend to experiences in forming attachments to the unborn child to which women are subject to the physical experiences of, and men to the more mental and visual evidence of in the form of antenatal screening programmes. Of note, are the difficulties in forming attachments to the unborn child following a previous death.

160

In particular, women in this study adopted varying coping strategies. For example in bartering with the baby to stay or by forming attachments once the previous child's gestational age of death has passed, thirty weeks, thirty four weeks. The following example suggests that detachment from the baby was paramount to a mother's emotional well being after the loss of her third child, a daughter:

R: At 20 weeks and the pregnancy, it was the hardest because of for every tweak...[pause upset]. It was the shortest one because for all that time we denied it was happening. We didn't want to get attached. It wasn't until we actually had the scan that right this is happening. We haven't changed the decorating in her room. I just can't bear to take it down it feels like a part of her...

Christina, mother of baby girl Ella-Leina (born at forty weeks, lived for thirteen days).

Within the previous narrative there is also the sense that guilt is felt owing to feelings of betrayal for having another child. By contrast other respondents' anxieties concerning their unborn child translated into increased monitoring both at home and hospital and more frequent antenatal screenings. These anxieties represent varying coping strategies within sub-plots the central component of which is the fear of the loss of the unborn child and a shift in respondents world view (taken for granted plot to no guarantee plot).

Further these sub-plots concerning detachment and then later attachment to the unborn child, also relate to the personhood of the baby within which ultrasound and biomedical technology contributes. The contradiction here is that these progressive techniques in the field of obstetrics were unable to intervene in a previous tragedy for these respondents. It is in this knowing that every eventuality has to be accounted for including the space to labour and birth with more privacy than on a labour ward. As has been previously noted these specific fears arose from previous experiences yet demonstrate that which is largely missing in the literature about subsequent pregnancies, which are women's emotional needs.

161

The following account is selected since it represents for many of the women interviewed, evidence of the fear and anxiety to which many experienced during another pregnancy:

R: One of my fears was that I was going to be left in a room and the heart beat would change and no one would know and the baby would be breech and nobody would know and it would be too late....One of the things I've got is that I don't want to be put in a room with a load of other women. It will be a hard, emotional time and it will bring quite a lot of memories back. I would like that personal time so if I want to sit and have a good cry I don't feel embarrassed with these four other women in the room with me.............
Sophia, mother of baby girl, Elen (born at twenty-four weeks, lived for two hours)

In keeping with Schott et al (2007), this account demonstrates that women in these circumstances require additional support. While this has been afforded to some respondents, it has been perceived as lacking for others, such that the following respondent felt the need to shout at a health professional during the labour and birth of her subsequent child:

R: I basically swore and basically told her to 'fuck off' out the room just as the registrar came in and he asked what's going on. I told him I think something's happening and she will not listen to me [attending midwife]. I can't bear her in the room she's been so rude to me, I've lost a baby plus I've had a miscarriage in between so I know when there is something happening He said, to her [midwife] "right you out the room and you lot get ready for breech vaginal delivery her feet are sticking out the cervix". What frightened me was that if I hadn't stood up to that midwife we might have lost Mia (subsequent child). That makes me feel very angry inside because that midwife could have been responsible for the death of my second daughter......
Trudy, mother of baby girl, Rose (stillborn at twenty-eight weeks).

While the previous account represents the anxiety and fear of a double tragedy it also implies less deference and trust in medical authority.

162

A lack of trust in others is borne of experience for some in the time following the birth of a subsequent child:

R:I know when I had Lexie (subsequent child) I cried solidly for six hours and not one person, not one of the midwives came to see me, to see what was up. I had a perfectly healthy baby and as far as I was concerned there should be nothing wrong but actually I was falling apart. I was an absolute wreck when she was born and I couldn't deal with her. I got a taxi and literally grabbed her and ran and I had to get out of the hospital. If someone had come in there and talked to me....They kept popping their head round the curtain and kept running away again it was absolutely horrendous. I just couldn't ask for help. You just need someone to come to you.... Continued

.....The thing I remember is in the bed opposite me there was obviously a girl who'd had a little boy and I had lost a little boy. All I can remember now is the grandmother saying what a lovely grandson you've given me and that just did it for me. I knew I had a healthy little girl, but........
Susie, mother of baby boy Billy (born at thirty-eight weeks, lived for nine hours).

Together these accounts demonstrate that certain behaviour in particular empathy and support is expected of medical professionals in a subsequent birth. Indeed the previous account reveals where this support could have been employed to greater effect. Yet it also suggests that having another child did not represent a sense of ease with the past since it was at this point that the mother unravelled (respondent's words). In her 'wreckage' are the faint words echoed by Langer (1991) earlier in this chapter that it was now her troubles were about to begin.

In this respect, the solution as that proffered by Cain and Cain (1964) earlier (replacement child) in this chapter is far from able to liberate this mother from her grief. This does not suggest that the subsequent child was unwanted: on the contrary, it was precisely because she was longed for which coincided with this respondent's grief for her previous child, and which culminated in her response to the birthing experience. This was a reality to which she related to further on in her biography of entering therapy for the first time in her life.

What this narrative and other accounts suggest is that what may be assumed to be the point of deepest chaos in their life, the central point of which is the death of a child, the continuous anxiety of a subsequent pregnancy and of the fear of loss of another child represents another form of chaos in the developing 'no guarantees' plot of the biography of respondents lives.

It is for this reason that though the experiences are similar the narratives need to be viewed in their own light and in terms of their sub-plots and in how their experiences came about. To this end they are of the same struggle: the past never leaves them, not even in the future. Their experiences remain embedded in their biography and within their sense of self.

Conclusion

In this first reading of the narratives embodied stories are presented as fragmented parts of a larger plot. The stories which follow are in themselves chaotic in their absence of a narrative order in that they are told as the respondent experiences their story in the interview. In making sense of these grieving voices, it can be seen that respondents have learned structures of narratives, metaphors, images and standards of what is and what is not socially appropriate to tell. It could be seen that where such stories are told in relation to the death of a child the sanctions which prohibit its re-telling are reinforced in some ways, and changed in others. Thus, it is the social context which affects which stories get told and how. Where these stories have been told, they represent the loss of the destination of respondent's mapped out lives which had previously guided them. Thus, they reveal some of the ways they have to learn to live differently in order to construct new perceptions of their relationship to the world.

These stories are anxiety provoking because in their telling the modern idea of remedy, progress and professionalism cracks to reveal vulnerability, futility and impotence. In so doing, stories do not simply describe the self, they are the self's way of being.

The self was described and shaped within the narratives by those experiences with others and with popular culture. It was these internalisations which led to confusion and to the subplot to men and women's stories which was about the taken for granted plot about pregnancy and birth.

While these experiences varied in relation to how they came about their effect was the same, one of grief and of a disrupted life course resulting in the 'no guarantees plot' of men and women's biography. This could be viewed in light of biomedical limitations which is as shocking to medicine as it is to men and women, since it represents challenges to modern ideas of progress.

These realities bring into focus the way discourses and specialist knowledge influence and shape how such experiences are defined. This in itself leads to great uncertainty following the death of respondents' children and of a deep rooted unpredictability in relation to life. Unlike the conventional narrative which has a past leading to a foreseeable future the death story is wrecked because its present is not what the past was supposed to lead up to, and the future is scarcely thinkable.

This is evident in the subsequent pregnancy narratives and to the idea that this would represent a sense of liberation from grief over the death of the previous child. I argued that this supposed freedom did not represent a break with the past: on the contrary it contributed to a sense of wreckage. It could be seen that one way out of this wreckage was for such self stories to be told.

This is about a dual reaffirmation because as the story is being narrated to the interviewer, it is being told to the self and, thus, reassured. In keeping with the suggestions of other heuristic researchers (Etherington, 2004:25; Frank, 1995:2), it was this research encounter which afforded attention to detail in the subsequent transcriptions and, thus, a reflexive approach to this research.

The following Chapter 6 will explore some of the ways in which men and women located themselves within their accounts of loss.

CHAPTER 6. Reading for the Voice of the 'I'

> *"I give myself verbal shape from another's point of view, ultimately, from the point of view of the community to which I belong. A word is a bridge thrown between myself and another."* (Volosinov, 1986:86)

Introduction

The previous chapter centred upon the relationship between the researcher and the person being interviewed and the way in which men and women contextualised their experiences in relation to loss and popular culture. This chapter explores some of the ways in which mothers and fathers locate themselves within their experiences of grief. The use of pronouns, narrative styles, contradictions and language are explored in relation to these experiences. Before turning to the narratives, I explain what it is to read for the voice of the 'I' in this chapter. While the voice of the 'I' can be found in feminist, legal theory and cultural and literary sources, there is no single agreement as to what this constitutes (Bakhtin 1984). For the purpose of this study, reading for the voice of the 'I' describes a way of presenting people's stories as told by them. This literally means searching for the personal pronoun (s) such as 'I', 'We' or 'You', and 'Other' respondents use in relation to talking about their experiences.

In this second reading of the transcripts, a case is made that 'I', represents the respondent at the centre of their story trying to make sense of the death of their child. It will be shown that in referring to the 'I', respondents expose the self as an individual who is isolated within their experiences of loss. In so doing, their grief is expressed within the confines of the story being told which is represented by silent pauses. For this reason, transcripts were listened to as well as read for, in order to capture the sense of aloneness with grief which permeated throughout men and women's narratives of death and loss.

167

This particular consideration of grief within the narratives, contrasts to respondents' reference to 'We', since it is an experience which is shared. This can be viewed in relation to respondents' reference to other people (spouses, family, and friends) within their narrative. Where these interactions are about a shared experience, respondents' reference to 'You' in their story represents their attempts to have an emotional distance from the story being told. It will be shown that metaphors are employed by narrators as a way of managing a difficult story to tell. These stories are challenging to tell precisely because they are about that which is difficult to comprehend – the death of a child in late modern times.

Yet within social interactions I argue that 'Other', is referred by respondents in relation to how they think others see them and which comprises an internal negotiation with the self. This way of thinking about a dialogic exchange can be found within cultural and literary orientations and with the ideas of Bakhtin (1984) and symbolic interactionists (Goffman, 1959; 1967). I argue, that these dialogic exchanges are reflexively subjective in that they represent a way for the self to experience another individuals' subjectivity from their own interior position. This is viewed in light of the way men and women in this chapter negotiate their status as a parent compared to socially available perceptions of motherhood and fatherhood.

This chapter concludes by suggesting that this second reading, the voice of the 'I' provides a way in which to elucidate how men and women give meaning to and contextualise their experience of the death of their children.

How the Mother Experiences Herself and the Death of Her Baby

In focusing on the use of pronouns in this second reading of the transcripts, I was able to note the changes in how respondents perceive and experience themselves (Mauthner and Doucet, 1998: 128). This enables men and women to speak for themselves rather than being spoken for. This serves to amplify the way in which the respondent presents themselves and pays attention to the difficulties respondents may be experiencing in telling their story either emotionally or intellectually. For example, the following account is useful to demonstrate a mother who is talking about her biographical self when using the 'I' yet seems uncertain of her status as a mother:

R:I was a mother and I didn't have a baby, it was like.... it was like that, it was like my identity had been taken away...............
Wynnie, mother of baby boy Bryn (stillborn at forty weeks).

This mother's sense of self was embedded in the relationship with her son. She continued to know herself as a mother but lost the self she knew in this relationship. In attempting to locate herself as a mother who is denied mothering, the respondent shifts from 'I' to analogous 'My'. This goes beyond signalling a change in how the respondent perceives herself: it represents the struggle to make sense of an experience. This particular brief part of a narrative is selected since it exemplifies a way of listening to transcripts. By creating the space between the way respondents narrate their story and researcher perception about the experience, they speak for themselves. Reading for the 'I' in this way exposes some of the ways women in this research perceive their status as a mother. In this regard, it reflects those issues which face both men and women in this study, when is a parent, a parent? Though these issues are pertinent for both the processes by which these statuses are claimed differ.

169

In the last chapter it was shown that a sense of fatherhood was deferred until a live subsequent child had been born. Conversely, the more physical work of labour and birth for many women respondents served as a rite of passage to motherhood:

R: People think your baby died, they don't think of the labour and how you are going to get them out. You have no preparation.... you go through the labour and I kept thinking it can't be right, it can't be right and then ... she's going to be dead but I still want to know if it's a girl or a boy and I still want to see her or him. That kind of kept me going. I refused pain relief because I wanted to experience it all......
Mel, mother of baby girl Bonnie (stillborn at thirty- nine weeks) .

R: One thing I always remember is that even though she was small I did feel her head coming out. I felt, I gave birth to her, even though there was no cry, I felt that. So again, she did exist I did feel that, that was quite good......
Trudy, mother of baby girl Rose (stillborn at twenty-eight weeks).

Though motherhood was a role which was socially unsustainable (especially for first time mothers), it was nevertheless a role which could be claimed privately. This is important in the context of social attitudes to ideas about women in relation to motherhood. Indeed, as Layne (2003: 59) argues, a woman is socially perceived as incomplete until she has borne a child. While this limiting view fails to consider the presence of the many socially varying familial households in Western societies for example, step families or adopted families and, thus, other ways of becoming a mother, it nevertheless represents for the majority of women in this thesis, a reality which they have to continuously negotiate socially. Indeed, with the first account (how did they think 'I' got her out?) the 'I' represents the making sense of the experience yet, it is also a way of comprehending other people's responses. As Bakhtin explains: *"we evaluate ourselves from the standpoint of others, and through others we try to understand and take into account what is transgredient to our own consciousness."* (1984:15)

Yet seeing our lives from the way others perceive us and from the consciousness of other people poses problems in claiming motherhood. For if others see us as non-mother, our sense of having achieved such status is challenged until it is a status that is claimed silently. Similarly, Bakhtin (1984:32) employs the analogy of a mirror by which we are able to reflect our *exterior* to others but not *ourselves.* This mirror of our exterior which we present in dialogic exchange provides a frame within which it is possible to assess the effect of our words upon others. This is evident in the first account where the physical work of labour and birth was perceived as a way of achieving the status of mother. Yet in social interaction it is a reflection which is betrayed by this mother's social network since it hints at a somewhat socially unacceptable rite, of which the only possible route is to produce a live child.

Bakhtin's consideration of the dialogic exchange is useful as its disciplinary orientation can be found in literary and cultural theory which while not sociological, align with symbolic interactionism and with the ideas of Goffman (1959). In particular, Goffman's interest in interaction stems from the premise that moral order is upheld in society by rituals. The expressive techniques used by individuals to maintain that order are 'dramarturgical', in that they are like those of actors. This performing is a form of social interaction between individuals which Goffman defined as symbolic interaction in that the self and others are referred to. While Bakhtin and symbolic interactionists differed in terms of their orientation, both refer to reflexive subjectivity. For Bakhtin, this means the self experiences another individuals' subjectivity and then returns to their own interior position. This can be seen with the last narrative account in testing out what can be said in front of others. This is critical to notions of becoming a parent for these women since it comes to define what is socially appropriate.

Indeed, for Turner (1982:232), pregnancy can be viewed as a temporary state which is 'betwixt and between fixed points of classification' and temporarily set apart from the structural arrangements of the culture. Similarly Stacey (1997:89), emphasises the transitional nature of pregnancy and as a borderline state in which there exists 'more than one but less than two' and a state of being in which the reassuring boundaries of self and other are lost (Stacey, 1997:89). It can be seen that this way of being ends following the birth and with the ritual confinement of mother and baby albeit for a few hours or days. It is a point where the pregnancy ends and the reintegration of the woman as a mother into the community begins. Though not all but some women experience congratulatory symbolic gestures, for example cards, and flowers, it represents a social ritual which defines new motherhood.

The difficulty for the majority of women interviewed is that there are no visible rites to incorporate the woman as mother. Their narrations are unable to incorporate such gestures because none were there. Their pregnancy and birth stories become death narratives and filled with condolence and awkward others. It is this sense of confusion which robs the women of their mother status and betrays the swollen belly that once held a precious child. This sense of 'I' sort of had a baby, and sort of had a child' is about making sense of the experience yet also contradicts the purpose of the hospital environment to which these events take place. It is this which represents a problem for women who lose their status as both mother and 'patient' within a hospital. This is in keeping with Lovell (1983), whose research about the support of women following stillbirths in London hospitals is discussed more widely in Chapter 3. As Lovell explains: *"it is as though hospitals seem to have no physical or psychological space for such a person, and the problem of a woman who seem to have no legitimate role was often solved by sending her home with what felt like indecent haste."* (1983: 757)

Lovell's arguments are in concert with some of the findings of this research and to which the following account has been selected to demonstrate some women's experiences in this thesis. It represents the dearth of a psychological and physical space in which to have such important moments with a child:

R: I just remember being in a chair holding Beth and watching her die, no curtains drawn. I remember other people being there and just people watching..... just people watching. We didn't have any privacy or dignity with you know I'm sat there. Is this really happening? Just in deep denial of it really just completely disempowered throughout. I thought they've banned fox hunting because it's barbaric and yet I've been in a hospital and felt like I'd been in a torture camp. I've lost my baby and am mentally and spiritually and physically annihilated and that's in a hospital that's supposed to provide care and look after you......

Paula, mother of baby girl Beth (born at forty weeks, lived for seventeen hours)

While this account varies in the way it came about (e.g. neonatal death) compared to others (prematurity or stillbirth) it nevertheless represents for several respondent's, a challenging experience in which they try to make sense. This is represented in the previous account with the shift from 'I' to 'We' to 'I'. There is the respondent as 'I' in trying to make sense of the situation to 'we' and of a shared grief with her husband, and then to the 'I' which represents the 'Me' attempting to make sense of the experience. In so doing the respondent remains at the centre of the experience which is isolating.

In the following account this sense of isolation is contextualised in relation to the death of a woman's son on the neonatal ward and in terms of this respondent's new status as a bereaved mother:

R I just had the worst feeling and I just dreaded the worst was going to happen. I just cried and cried and said I think Jack [baby who died] is giving up I think he is leading us up the garden path. As we were having that conversation he [baby Jack] gave up. We got there [neonatal unit from side room] and they were resuscitating him and they were keeping him alive. The doctor said: 'he's not going to make it we would like your permission to stop' and I said: 'no don't' stop keep going'....I don't know how much time passed, he came back in [doctor attending to baby Jack] and he said: 'we really need your permission to stop.' We have been resuscitating him for twenty minutes now.' I don't know how we decided but we said: 'OK'. We actually gave him permission which is not a nice thing to do is it? And then I held him for the first time and the last time. And then that's when you're a bereaved parent and off you go then really isn't it?
Selena, mother of baby boy Jack (born at thirty-eight weeks, lived for two days).

This account provides an example of how the respondent, Selena attempts to make sense of the experience by stabilising her position (I) in the story which is isolated. The second person 'You' (You're) is employed and suggests a shift in herself and an emotional distancing. Reference to 'I' then to 'Other' serves to justify a course of action whereby the doctor has tried for twenty minutes to resuscitate this baby boy and asked for permission to stop which was reluctantly granted by the parents.

In both previous accounts reference to others appears as a means of comparison for the respondent's own experiences. This generalised otherness also suggests an internal complex negotiation of events. Similarly, for Holdsworth and Morgan (2007:403), this otherness provides a way to conceptualise and understand processes of comparison and judgement and is an internal conversation with the self. This idea of other then concerns respondents' reflexive practices which connect to symbolic interactionism, in that the social interaction which takes place between people, takes account of the self and others.

174

In this reflexive subjectivity the previous account further demonstrates where one voice is caught between two voices which articulate opposing positions and different ways of assessing the situation. This relates to expectations about the respondent as a mother and willing her son to live and of the expectations about the doctor to discontinue in aspirating her dying child. Not least, it represents an experience which has no discourse by which to refer, other than to which the doctor recommends, medicine. This internalisation of the attitude and actions of others in narratives reflects a dialogue between competing voices, such they may 'drown' respondents' own.

For example, in the following account, the mother in remaining silent made room for these 'other voices', and withheld her emotions:

R: My mother-in-law was incredibly upset about losing Melody and Joy and I used to feel angry with her because she was taking away my role as the main grieving person. She'd be in tears and I would be sitting there not crying and thinking that made me a terrible mother because I wasn't crying and she was. I couldn't cry in front of her. I couldn't cry in front of my parents either. I could cry in front of Ian [husband] at home on our own but I couldn't share it with other people…
Ruth, mother of baby girls Melody and Joy (born at twenty-seven weeks, lived for two hours).

In listening for the respondent's voice in the previous account she is speaking of herself in the first person 'I', and articulates her position in relation to the other actors within the story. These relational voices carry ways of being in a relationship which is to be emotionally silent and existing in sufferance since like the language; the respondent is embedded within this web of relationships. It can be seen that the voice is eloquent yet in pain. In talking about relationships with others we get to hear the frustration and the anguish. Moreover, the experience is reduced to a topic, thus, denying the story's main condition which is the fact that the parent has experienced the death of her children.

175

It is a story which someone (mother-in-law), interrupts which represents the interruption in the respondent's life. It not only describes what has happened, it is an interrupted story since the responses of the mother-in-law disrupts one story line in order to establish another.

This digression brings into awareness the conditions by which the respondent is able to express her emotions and the means of performing or engaging in them. It as though they want no further intrusion.

With this particular narrative even the most benevolent intention remains an intrusion and, thus, an interruption. The narrative then, is an attempt to restore order that the interruption fragmented and to a different kind of purpose. This attempt continues when the mother employs metaphors:

R: It's a strange beast grief isn't it? You will read a story and there is something in there which strikes a chord and you sort of ... it brings everything back to you. It's like physical healing, the scar tissue gradually builds up and it heals over but sometimes old scars get knocked and they hurt, it's the same with emotions as well. I wacked my knee in the swimming pool years and years ago, but if I knock it at the right angle it's still excruciating and it's the same thing. If you read something or see something on the wrong day at the wrong time, just in that not quite right frame of mood it can bring everything back with a vengeance.....

Ruth, mother of twin baby girls Melody and Joy (born at twenty-seven weeks, lived for two hours).

The previous account demonstrates how metaphors work in bereavement narratives by drawing upon another embodied experience of injury to describe grief thereby establishing another story line.

This use of metaphor is a way of making sense of the world in a culturally meaningful way by emotionally distancing the self from the story. Further, it exposes the differentiation between public and private accounts of grief. Similarly, Cornwell (1984:11-17), in writing about his analysis of health and illness narratives, suggests that 'public accounts' are culturally normative and produce common sense responses which are safe as they do not involve disclosure and the reopening of painful emotions.

176

By contrast, 'private accounts' involve disclosure and the re-opening of potentially harmful emotions. This suggests that mother in the first account was unable to cry in front of her relatives as this was too distressing. It was only with her husband that she felt safe enough to express emotion.

As several of the women interviewed spoke about their experiences of grief and loss, they often (as in the previous account), switched between pronouns within the same paragraph because public and private accounts were inadequate in describing their experiences:

R: It's very sad you know I can wake up one morning and feel absolutely crap. You don't know, you know why you do, you know why but you can feel crap and you can look after the other children you have and you can go up to the primary school and someone can say 'oh hi how are you?' And if you turn round and say, I'm feeling absolutely crap actually.....I miss Katie (baby who died). They are going to think Oh God! You can't even say that anymore. I can say it to my friend if I'm having a bit of a roughie day. I still get quite cross really.........

Sandy, mother of baby girl Katie (stillborn at forty weeks).

R: I don't worry so much about what people think of me it's how I see myself and that I've lost a baby and that will always be a part of me that I carry around. You think four years down the line how am I going to be dealing with this? You do because you don't have much choice, the sun keeps rising everyday..............

Briony, mother of baby boy Samuel (stillborn at forty-three weeks).

These accounts both demonstrate the difficulty in telling the listener an aspect of experience. The 'I' in trying to make sense of what it is to live each day without their children is an attempt to dissociate themselves from the experiences with the use of 'You' to convey an emotional distancing. Where these examples demonstrate the problematic use of the pronoun, they reveal the impact of the dialogic exchange in social interaction and respondents' reflexive subjectivity. These exchanges become internalised and silence voices since they set in place what is socially appropriate and to whom reference to feelings in relation to the child can be shared. This has particular relevance to the social construction of motherhood, a status it is argued, which acts as a relatively solid and reliable source of self and identity.

For Schilling (1997:178) these social positions allow men and women to make sense of what is real and meaningful about their embodied selves and the world around them.

The problem for men and women in this research however, is in attempting to contextualise their experiences in relation to what is left of their embodied selves which gives rise to confusion. Indeed, the cultural construction of motherhood and fatherhood in respondent's eyes at least, represents a discontinuity with their status and represents an ideological crisis. These ideas have been considered in relation to women in this chapter, and to which I now turn to that of the men and their experiences. Particular attention is given to the emotional significance of their loss in relation to their sense of ambivalence concerning fatherhood, since this was a strong theme throughout mens' narratives

How the Father Experiences Himself and Death of His Baby

Several authors (Coltrane, 2007; Murphy and Hunt 1997; Worth, 1997), suggest that fatherhood represents social practices and expectations that are institutionalised within culture. This can be viewed in light of attending ultra sound scans and antenatal appointments with a pregnant partner. It is these practices which for these authors, add to the sense of fatherhood and changing identity and to bonding between a father and his unborn child. This has relevance to the symbolic significance of the baby for fathers in this study.

The following account demonstrates the ambivalence a father felt about the physical presence of his baby and trying to identify the unique relationship he had already formed with this child:

R:Holding my son, you know. I don't know if I would have done that, you know, I don't know if I would've spent time looking at his body if those people around me hadn't have suggested that that was a good idea you know. Um, [pause] um, so now it's obviously a moment that I treasure. It's an important, very important, physical experience. Purely on a physical level kind of I'd kind of go, this is an empty vessel, a body that I have had you know have had a hand in creating. In one way this is not my son because he is gone…

178

..But, this is something physical; this is something like on a kind of animal level that I need to have this close physical experience. Um, so that was important. I think I only held him once at that immediate afterwards……

Karl, father of baby boy Bryn (stillborn at forty weeks).

The 'I' is referred to considerably in this narrative part and represents the respondent at the centre of his isolating experience in holding his child. It is a sense making story in which the father tries to define between the physical and the existential, the telling of which occurs with little reference to others despite the significance of 'other peoples' encouragement to hold his son. His sense of fatherhood is exposed by reference to the physical and primeval need to hold his child and his hand in creating the vessel that is the body of his child.

While Karl's account demonstrates that fatherhood is defined as a physical contribution and, thus, an emotional and biological link between a male parent and his child, the following account demonstrates the emotional significance of loss for other men

R: It was absolutely devastating. The days afterwards, it was dark, miserable and raining, we barely wanted to eat anything. Each day we wanted to go in and see our daughters… I know after we lost Melody and Joy I've never been suicidal and I hope I never am but it's the closest I can imagine being. You almost got to the stage where you didn't care and then you think what is the point of anything, of absolutely anything. If we had a child already that would have been different you've got a reason to live. I believe the whole point of life is to procreate. When you are looking over that abyss of not having a child it really becomes a horrendous abyss…..

Ian, father of baby twin girls, Melody and Joy (born at twenty-seven weeks, lived for two hours).

This father's shift from 'We' to 'I' suggests both a grief that was shared with his wife, (the mother of his twin girls) and a strong sense of his own personal grief as the father. In being less certain in talking about himself,

179

Ian shifts from the first person (I) to the third person (You), with the 'You' representing an emotional distancing that is necessary to disclose a feeling which is wounding (how he felt at the time of loss compared to how he feels now). Indeed, the whole point of life for this father was to have children and nothing else compared to achieving fatherhood. This concurs with Coltrane's (2007:448),study about fatherhood where male respondents rank marriage and children among their most precious goals. Similarly, Layne (2003:152), contends that while women's role in reproduction is more extensive, men suffer a sense of loss such that their sexual identity may be affected. Indeed, the previous account demonstrates a sense of powerlessness and of a sense of self which is threatened.

It is this direct threat to this sense of fatherhood that I turn to the words of Victor Frankl (2006) to expose the vulnerability of the respondent's position: *"It is a peculiarity of man that he can only live by looking to the future – sub specie aeternitatis. And this is his salvation in the most difficult moments of his existence, although he sometimes has to force his mind to the task."*(2006:73) Indeed, this Ian's reference to suicide and the pointlessness of life is viewed in stark contrast to his purpose for being, which is to procreate. This sense of hopelessness in relation to creating life is represented by looking at a future which is nothing more than a 'horrible abyss'. While eloquent and articulate, this reading and listening of the narrative revealed some of the way respondents adopted a wandering pronoun (I/We/You) in their narrative when they were struggling with something to say. Similarly, in the following example, a father talks about finding a location which best expressed how he felt following the loss of his son:

R: I read up a lot on people's experiences and for me I found the poetry the most poignant. Angela [wife] has read lots of books. I would find that too much I don't want to keep reading about people's losses. I did to see how it compared but the poetry I think was the most closest. Sometimes I think you can say things in a poem that you can't really express any other way. There was a couple of them, well one and it's called the grief club. It goes on… you are member of this club that nobody applies to join….
Andy, father of baby boy, Ollie (born at forty weeks, lived for twelve days).

The movement from 'I' to You/We in the previous account provides an example of a shared link to a club and a place where others have experienced such deaths. It is a narrative which reveals the beginning of a journey symbolic of loneliness and isolation and towards a distancing from others because it is too much to bear. What feels safest in this private narrative is poetry, and it is this way of finding meaning which exposes an anguished memory trying to find the words which are consonant with his existence as a bereaved father.

Reading for the voice of the 'I' in the previous and other accounts of loss has served as a constant reminder to establish the authenticity of the voice before responding to the text. In this regard the narratives unfold both visually and by listening to voices which are heard.

To this end, the utility of employing the voice relational method in this study has proved valuable in considering how men and women struggle to find meaning as they shift between notions of I/You, Self/Other and (Mother/Father/Other). This sense of shift in the narrative and fluidity in identity is further considered by exploring respondents' narrative styles.

Narrative Styles

The use of the pronoun in respondents' narratives has been described in relation to how the mother and father see themselves and their experiences. By paying closer attention to the reading it is possible to discern and expose the familiarity by which the respondent tells his or her story. Similarly, Layne (2003:6-7), reveals how in her own account of pregnancy losses, storytelling involves revisiting one's narrative as new data emerges. Instead of a single narrative many stories are produced, revisited and rehearsed as a means of attending to the damage created by loss. This suggests that as responses to the loss change over time so does the way in which men and women tell their story.

Following interviews, several women disclosed that telling their story had been emotionally depleting, yet also cathartic. Of note is one respondent's sense of relief about feeling less censured than when in other social interactions and it is this which was powerful in telling her story.

While fathers' spent time in telling their story and in some instances held longer interviews than mothers, they did not reveal the same sense of catharsis or tiredness as mothers. Yet most were able to express emotion and in some instances cry when narrating.

Other stories sounded more rehearsed as though they had been told on several occasions. These tended to be narrated by respondents whose babies died several years ago. This is explained by continuous or previous attendance at support group meetings where they would be expected to share their experiences on several occasions, especially when new members arrived.

Further examples demonstrate the way in which a story was reframed from the first storytelling at interview to the focus group which occurred several months later. During the first interview the following respondent expressed her anxiety and her inability to trust life in the same way again following the death of her baby girl, Lucy:

R: Since Lucy died I have been on constant red alert, occasionally I switch to Amber and be a bit more chilled but at the drop of a hat I'm back to red alert again – literally waiting on edge all the time. That's why I'm so anxious and stressed. It's no way to live your life because I don't want to be like that for the rest of my life. But at the moment I'm not prepared to go to green and think that everything is alright and everything could be alright……

Isobel, mother of baby girl Lucy (stillborn at forty weeks).

The previous mother's overwhelming sense of anxiety following the death of her baby is repeated again in a focus group which occurred several months later......

R: I'm not prepared to be relaxed and to feel everything's OK .I'm frightened that if I do, something will go wrong again and I won't be prepared for it so I'm constantly trying to be prepared for something going wrong even though it probably won't........
Focus group 2, Isobel, mother of baby girl Lucy (stillborn at forty weeks).

Similarly, another woman described the impact of loss in an interview:

R: I just felt completely and utterly detached as though no one could possible reach me now. It's impossible to know how to deal with it; you just have to do things you have to. I lost a lot of weight, I was thin as a rake and I couldn't sleep.....
Briony, mother of baby boy Samuel (stillborn at forty- three weeks).

Which she reiterated again at a later date...

R: I still don't sleep particularly well. I think after the first few months that is when you really need the support because all of a sudden physically you are mended but all the details come back to you... all the haunting details. Even now... it can't have all happened it must have been a nightmare...
Focus group 4, Briony, mother of baby boy Samuel (stillborn at forty-three weeks).

These accounts suggest that respondents' narratives were specifically chosen as a public account of loss and a part of their story they were comfortable in telling (Cornwell 1984: 204). Similarly the process of being asked to discuss issues as part of a focus group prompts the disclosure of a public account which carries little risk of harm compared to the more private telling of the story (interview) which can re-open emotional wounds of loss. The narrative styles within these accounts demonstrate the fluidity in one compared to a static story in another and which exposes the rawness of both women's experiences.

There is the sense that the anxiety felt by one mother will prevail throughout her life and, thus, her story will never change. Conversely in the second account there is a disbelief about how awful life was and a glimmer of hope albeit small, that the way she experiences herself and tells her story may improve.

These narratives were selected since they represent other respondents' references to hope as well as despair which are at odds in their telling. This exposed contradictions in their story and even within the same paragraph which is considered in relation to men and womens experiences of loss.

Contradictions

There is a sense of conflict and uncertainty which permeates throughout respondent's narratives which are exposed by the contradictions in the telling of the story. For example, the account given below exposes the inner conflict when considering existential issues in relation to a first child who died (Lucy) and the reality of her life with her subsequent child, Evie:

R: I used to wish myself dead and be with Lucy but when you've got your other little one it's like they've both got hold of each arm and they're pulling you each way, I wanna be with Lucy [baby who died] and I wanna be with Evie [child born after baby who died]. Sometimes you resent the fact that you can't be with both of them. If for just one day I could be with the both of them and have my two little girls with me that would be so great, just for one day and then I would let her go again, I wouldn't but you know what I mean. It's awful I think I've got to wait until I die before I get to see her but then if I die it means I have to leave Evie and other people that I love and people that love me so it really tugs on you sometimes as to which way......

Isobel, mother of baby girl Lucy (stillborn at forty weeks)

The previous example demonstrates the recurring discrepancy between the 'I' which emphatically states that she wants to be with her daughter who has died and also with her second daughter who is living. These mixed sentiments are critical in discerning between a desire to die and a desire to live in relation to the impact of the death of a child.

184

There is an aspect of uncertainty about her own identity as the mother to a living as well to a dead child and the meaning of the loss which is exhibited (e.g. I wanna be with Lucy and I wanna be with Evie).

What this account demonstrates is the way some men and women experience difficulties in adjusting to a lost relationship because the nature of the death (stillbirth or neonatal death) excludes them from sharing their experiences (other than a support group), and therefore being able to make sense of it.

Other contradictions which are present within respondent's accounts expose the emotional impact of loss which while similar in intensity, varies in terms of how they came about. For example, several respondents talked about knowing or feeling that something was wrong with their unborn child at varying gestational ages. Despite these embodied symptoms the sense of shock, despair and sadness are one and the same in these accounts. The following example describes a mother's embodied knowing in relation to bleeding at an earlier stage of gestation:

R: There was a feeling through most of it that it wasn't quite going to work itself out well. I had another bit of bleeding later on but again not very much so we had another scan. I just sat on the bed and said I just can't see this baby happening I couldn't see it, it was really weird. As time went on you can feel it kicking and I was thinking this is going to be great, if it was a girl. It was fine, and it was I wasn't really taking much notice of the kicking and at the same time thinking I couldn't see the pregnancy happening. But yeah it is going on you are in a sort of cocoon of security you know and I just went along. You get to a certain point you just don't think anything is going to go wrong.....
Lou, mother of baby girl, Marie-Rose (stillborn at twenty-seven weeks).

At twenty-seven weeks, the mother in the previous account went for a routine check up. The midwife could not find a heartbeat and the baby's death was confirmed by an ultrasound scan...

R: I just remember screaming immediately. It was just like one of those weird animal like cries that you don't know is inside you until it happens.....

This contradictory retelling of a story reflects other respondent's accounts of hope and fears in relation to their embodied selves.

From the same account, Lou later went on to write this poem in dedication to her daughter....

You were not pretty, yet you were beautiful
You did not breathe, yet you had life
You were not meant to be, but you had meaning
I never held you, but you were mine.

The poem is included here since it demonstrates the way several respondents narrated their sense of loss in relation to their experiences through poetry. Again, while each differs in how the deaths of their children came about, they nevertheless imply that the impact of their loss is great and is of a grief which is long lasting.

While there is not sufficient room within this thesis to include all of men and women's poetry, the previous example provides a way in which to elucidate some of the ways respondents find ways of expressing their grief. The poetry presented here came about in relation to the respondent's hospital birthing experience. In an interview with this mother, she referred to the response of staff who discouraged her from seeing her daughter and who later lost the one photo that was taken of her child. Thus, the respondent's reference to 'not being pretty enough' is linked to the responses and actions of professionals. As Lou explains:

R: You just think what have I given birth to? you know not having a photo, not being recommended to view the baby was just, was just, gosh you know. You know it's a baby, you know it's a human baby, you know it's not a monster. It's just those little words can be really damaging you know. I wasn't really encouraged to remember it or talk about it afterwards, it was very silent.....
Lou, mother of baby girl, Marie-Rose (stillborn at twenty-seven weeks).

The perceived actions of others in this narrative add to the contradiction in the story and served to confer some form of spoiled identity upon the baby. Thus, the women in this instance as well as having a dead baby, had an imperfect baby and as such viewed herself as a double deviant (Lovell, 1983: 756). This ambiguous state of Mother or Other also emanated from the narratives of parents who do not have the words or the expression to describe their embodied experiences.

Not Having the Words to Express the Experience

For Lambeck (1996: 243 - 249), trauma is an "intrinsic part of self hood" and given the sense of trauma that the death of a baby can create in the self, the 'identity-building act' of remembering is crucial. Yet the death of a baby poses a number of challenges in terms of memorialising with others because they were a child few people knew. In the following accounts such silences represent wounded grieving selves immersed in shock. There are no words; only the struggle in trying to find them. The following narrative provides an example of this, as one mother attempts to retell her story and recall her memory of events immediately following the birth and death of her daughter in hospital:

R: I was odd at the time Kerry [researcher] like I didn't know. I was just back in this 'echoee' bubble where everything was like slow motion and people were just walking in, like in those films as you watch people walk out and someone would come in and be taking photographs of Abbie. She just came in and dropped the negatives film disc thing beside on the bedside table and said: 'don't lose that'.
Tina, mother of baby girl Abbie (stillborn at forty weeks).

For another mother recalling events several years later....

R: There's no rhyme or reason to it half the time something just triggers it off and that is quite scary. Even now that occasionally happens to me something just triggers......
Susie, mother of baby boy, Billy (born at thirty-eight weeks, lived for nine hours).

187

These accounts were selected since they demonstrate some of the ways respondents' had difficulty in finding the words for their experience at varying stages of their narration. In so doing, they expose the vulnerability of women who have little or no control over events and circumstances, not even in the years that follow. They are in a sense, chaotic narratives since they are defined as being as part of a film, the script of which they did not write. There is the effort to reassert some sense of order in this story which fails at the 'rhyme or reason', precisely because there is none. This reveals the lack of contingency that is both difficult and 'scary' to accept but is reluctantly accepted nonetheless. Moreover, such living is viewed as inevitable since there is always the 'trigger' which act as the fear point of the story which is the fear of reliving the death of a child.

This struggle in telling a story represents the difficulty in living with loss more generally. It reflects a lack of discourse in relation to the death of a baby and in trying to find empathic interlocutors. This concerns the following respondent as he reflects upon his own fears and difficulties in expressing loss with others in the interview:

R: There was someone at our SANDS group whose husband didn't want to get involved in any of these groups and seemed to get over it, then years later they were down at the Zoo and suddenly he just burst into tears and he couldn't go any further and he had to be taken home. For some reason, it hit him all that time later at what seems like some total random point of time. Hearing that maybe I think maybe that is what is going to happen to me. One of them at SANDS said it had happened to them nine years ago and that was a bit disconcerting. I thought Christ I'm not going to be coming here for nine years. I would hope that by then....

Andy, father of baby boy Ollie (born at forty weeks, lived for twelve days).

Reference to another bereaved father in this narrative is representative of two adjacent worlds which intrude on each other since it evokes an anxiety which reflects a larger issue.

It is about a dread which is exposed as it is in reference to a collapsed man who broke down which is ultimately what the respondent fears.

It is a story of the consequences of loss: it knows a truth in a way that other people don't know it, because they are the ones that have lived it.

Indeed, what this account reveals are those of the narratives more generally. Though they are stories about the death of a child, how they are told and in what way vary. This is because men and women are trying to convey their story in a meaningful way. The genesis of the problem in struggling to find the words to define the experience emanate from previous audiences (family, friends and others) where they have been tested out.

It can be seen that the difficulty others face in listening to these narratives reflects an active fear of avoidance since it forces us to consider that which we are unable to control, fate.

In this context, the death of a baby is a social problem because of its potential to challenge people's sense of what is meaningful about their embodied selves and the world around them (Schilling, 1997: 179). The deaths of respondents' children cannot be conveyed in a way which is plainly factual or without emotion. They are at times told from a distance or with silent pauses representing as they do the anguish and the frustration that the story they are trying to tell drives off the audience they seek to capture. In these social interactions lessons have been learnt. A reluctance to share stories does not imply a preference to be silent with others. On the contrary, it is because such stories are silenced that these bereavement narratives are rich in their context in this thesis.

Conclusion

The second reading of the data enabled close attention to be paid to how men and women experienced their selves and identities in relation to the birth and death of their babies. They serve to elucidate how they continue to experience themselves in the broader social contexts in which they live. Reading and paying close attention to the 'I', represented an attempt to hear the person voice her or his sense of agency whilst taking into account the social location of the person who is telling their story (Mauthner and Doucet, 1998: 130). This served to expose the multi-layered voices within a narrative and illuminate both mother's and father's experiences and their subjective perception of subsequent events.

Foregrounding parents words provided the location in which a particular part of the story is placed and also exposed the difficulty some men and women have in narrating their re-telling a traumatic event. Some men and women provided an account that remained fixed in time, while others were more rehearsed.

The different use of pronouns and narrative styles demonstrated the changing relationship to the experience of loss and to themselves, especially where subsequent children had been born. These accounts draw upon public and private accounts of loss both of which while useful, are unable to fully explain why gendered accounts of loss differ in their expression. Such differing accounts deconstruct notions of homogeneity in responses to grief. There are men and women able to find the words to describe their grief, while others struggle to tell their story and employ metaphor as a means of defining their experiences. Contradictory accounts of loss expose the complexity in finding meaning, while the use of metaphor suggests that the experience of loss is embedded with other experiences over the life course which are familiar and viewed as part of the historical track of a men and women's biography.

CHAPTER 7. Reading for the Relationships

Introduction

In the previous two chapters the narratives were read for the overall stories and for respondents' different voices. In the third reading of these narratives, attention is given to listening for how men and women spoke about their interpersonal relationships - with their partners, their relatives, their children, health professionals and the broader social networks in which they worked and lived and how these relationships have influenced the way they have coped with their experience of the death of their baby. It is argued that the interpretations that each parent is able to draw upon to make sense of the loss will be affected by the beliefs and attitudes both in the wider culture and within various sub-cultural groups.

In this third reading I attend to the way respondents' talk about their relationships with others and note the struggles and ways in which they are empowered to express their grief. I begin by exploring respondents relationships with their partners and question normative assumptions about gendered emotional responses to loss. I argue that the social and cultural milieu to which these mythologies belong do not fit with respondents' realities. I distinguish between narratives which become distorted by gender stereotypes and those which are more harmonious and empowering because of their demonstrative emotionality on behalf of men. It will be shown that the present confusion in respondents narratives emanate from that which they know about relationships through experience and what is socially constructed and this is why parents struggle in some relationships.

I also consider the influence of other influential relationships in respondents' lives and explore the presence of surviving siblings and relatives. I expose the vulnerabilities in those relationships and their consequences.

I do this by listening for the self silencing within respondents' narratives and capitulation to a debilitating cultural script which are marked by respondents' reference to buried feelings which manifest in confusion, uncertainty and dissociation from relationships.

It will be shown that these particular relationships provide either opportunities for coping with grief or emotional distancing and exclusion.

This sense of confusion extends to relationships with health professionals due in part to institutional and varying professional approaches to loss, which reflect practices that reinforce cultural norms and social values surrounding stillbirth and neonatal death. In so doing, it exposes a medical discourse which reinforces those statuses assigned to men and women. Moreover, respondents' accounts reveal that their bereavement role is placed in a modern narrative of social control since medicine cannot place the bereaved in any other narrative other than that which reflects a social hierarchy. To this end, I conclude by arguing that both institutions and individual listeners steer the bereaved towards certain narratives since those which are more resonant with respondents' lives are difficult to witness and contemplate. These particular barriers to emotionality mean that men's and women's bereavement stories remain unheard until they seek mutually supportive relationships with others, within a sub-culture of bereaved parents.

I begin exploring respondents' relationships with their spouse and consider how they posit themselves within the experience. This brings into focus the couples' everyday experiences; a perception of how things should be and how they are currently configured and experienced.

Relationship with Partners

Rubin (2007: 322) argues that the differences in the psychology of men and women are born of a complex interaction between society and the individual. At the social level is the rending of thought and feeling that is a part of western thought. Thought is defined as the ultimate good and assigned to men; feeling, considered at best a problem, has fallen to women. Thus, the concept of the 'rational man - hysterical woman' cultural script is so firmly and socially entrenched that it is perceived as a natural and scientific truth. The following narrative demonstrates what is assumed to be a gender specific mode of expression of grief. It is told by a mother who is talking about her style of coping compared to her husband's:

R: I think he wanted to keep a stiff upper lip and be strong and supportive for me. In a way I'm glad that he was but I also wish he'd showed his feelings a bit more. I don't know if he knows this but I did catch him once sobbing in the shower and I just left him in there. I just wanted to read books, and surf the internet and read poems and look at book after book, after book. I got on so many websites all over the place and read everything and talked to people. He just didn't find any help or comfort in doing that. He chose to get a hacksaw and cut off all the limbs of the trees in the garden. Men are from Mars and women are from Venus that sort of thing, there's no right way to grieve...................
Claire, mother of baby girl Lara (stillborn at forty-one weeks).

Whilst the husband's grief is active and symbolic of physical masculinity and expression, there is a need to urge caution. The previous narrative states that the husband did cry which suggests an intense grief which was felt and expressed albeit more privately. This suggests that the emotional magnitude of the loss is as great as for this father as it is for the mother. This suggests that social expectations of behaviour may create gendered norms and as a consequence men are burdened with controlling their emotions. Indeed, the husband's deployment with the hacksaw and more private moment in the bathroom are reflective of this 'solitary expressivism'.

For Seidler (2004) concealing emotional pain and being dependable is often viewed as a masculine trait. Yet women in this study demonstrate a degree of emotionality and organisation around the death usually associated with men in the literature:

R: I went into practical mode and said we've got to arrange the funeral and we've got to do this and we've got to do that. Since then it's been the other way round. He's been the one who's practical, he's the one who has gone back to work...
Briony, mother of baby boy Samuel (stillborn at forty-three weeks).

R: We went to bed late and I can remember waking in the early hours [pause tears] and it kind of hit me [tears] in the early hours and I just came down and made a cup of tea [pause tears]. The next day it was just keeping busy. We were total opposites. I just surprised myself how I was. I'm normally the one that can't cope with things and cry and stuff. Alan [husband] was just in bits he kept getting up every two minutes, but I was sort of the strong one and I had a job to do and that was to bury my daughter...............
Sophia, mother of baby girl Elen (born at twenty-four weeks, lived for two hours).

These narratives were selected since they reflect the activities of several women around the death of their child. For these women the funeral represented something that they could do for their child. This compares to some of the men in this study who preferred their partners to organise the funeral:

R: When it came to organising the funeral, Wynnie [partner] did everything, it was really important for her to do those things and I wasn't interested in the slightest you know. Um, she [Wynnie] went and got him [baby Bryn] from the hospital and brought him home which I found very difficult again, but I knew that it was important for her and to people who hadn't seen him................
Karl, father of baby boy, Bryn (stillborn at forty weeks).

This account exposes the emotional magnitude of the loss for some men and why they find it difficult to engage in these funerary activities.
There is a sense of tension in undertaking this role as though it is expected of him compared to the challenging reality that he simply can't, it is too painful.

194

This suggests, as with the other narratives that there is no one universal gendered grieving pattern which can explain perceived differences in the way mothers and fathers grieve and cope with their loss. Yet as Chapter 2 demonstrates, differences exist to the extent that they create tension in a relationship. The following narrative has been selected as a demonstration of the difficulties some partnerships endure:

R: Unfortunately my husband is the worst of the lot of them for talking about it. I ended up going to counselling. Obviously I had a big problem with my husband and the resentment I held towards him and she said you have just got to accept that is just the way that he is and put up with it so I did, for years. Then suddenly I got to the point where.....
I can't do this anymore, I cannot ... I am angry with him and that anger has been simmering away for years and it was beginning to affect our marriage. My resentment was starting to come back whereas I had managed to keep it suppressed for a number of years. Suddenly it was all coming back....................
Susie, mother of baby boy, Billy (born at thirty-eight weeks, lived for nine hours).

In the previous account the death of a child has brought about uncertainty and instability within a relationship such that resentment and anger is felt many years later. While many respondents have discussed the tension within their relationship following loss, the majority of respondents did remain together. Of the two respondents whose relationships did break down, it was not possible to discern the underlying cause without causing further distress in interviews.

In contrast to other men and women's experiences in this research, other respondent's discussed some of the ways in which the death of their child had brought about closeness in their relationship:

R: We've been very lucky. I've heard of couples who have fallen apart. In our case it hasn't been the case. It is corny but it has made us stronger together. Again people react differently in different circumstances. I think you just have to get through things. I used to come home and we used to hold each other and cry just all the time........
Ian, father of twin girls Melody and Joy (born at twenty-seven weeks, lived for two hours)

These varying narratives are significant in that they challenge the general representation of grieving men and women more widely in popular culture. Similarly Dermott (2008:69) in writing about fatherhood suggests that the idea of fathers being less affected by the death of their child compared to their partners derives, in part, from representations of grief within the media. For example, Dermott (2008) argues that news stories are more likely to contain images of an inconsolable mother compared to a father when the death of a child is reported upon by the popular press. Further, in Chapter 2, research was quoting as showing that men are less affected by the death of their child than women (Vance et al, 1995). Yet the previous two chapters in this thesis showed that men's sense of loss is as great as that of women in this research. This is partly explained by technological innovation such as ultrasound scans and greater involvement in pregnancy which serves to create a sense of fatherhood for men.

A lack of research concerning men's grief has led in part, to a wider cultural misunderstanding about masculinity and bereavement. Moreover unlike motherhood and fatherhood of live children, relationships between bereaved parents lack their own representation in the public sphere.
For Thompson (1997) gendered emotional responses to loss: *'is a question of degree and emphasis, rather than a simple either or.'* (1997:82) Thompson's particular focus upon emotionality within relationships takes note of the subtleties in expressing grief.

What differs in this regard between the men and women in this research are the displays of emotion and the location of their expression. It is because of this misrecognition that men are perceived as unemotional, leading to tension and in some instances breakdown in a relationship.

While these familial systems of communication are much discussed in the literature, the impact of surviving children on bereaved parents' loss is largely ignored (Segal et al, 1995). A discussion on children in the family is significant to this study since they mediate men's and women's responses to loss.

196

Relationship with Surviving Children in the Family

While the death of children represents challenges in a relationship, some men and women face adapting to the changes in the way they parent their surviving children. For example, Dyregrov (2008) in his research with grieving children noted that the sense of disequilibrium parents feel in their inner life could extend to their parenting. While this is disconcerting, there is a dearth of research pertaining to this issue, particularly in relation to death following stillbirth or neonatal death. Indeed, while the sense of grief and loss was similarly described for all respondents in this study, the way in which they parented the relationship with their surviving child varied. It is useful to turn to Schiff (1997: 83–84) as a bereaved mother and as an author of grief and loss, since she maintains that one of the most difficult challenges following the death of a child is to continue to be a parent to surviving children.

Similarly, Rosenblatt's (2000), study of bereaved parents following the death of a child, suggests that there was a distancing between surviving children and their parent as they were either preoccupied with their grief or wanted to protect the children from their own emotions. For example, the following account demonstrates the difficulty in parenting a surviving child when preoccupied by the grief over the death of a son:

R: In the early days I felt resentment towards Jacob [surviving child]. I wasn't unkind or anything I was just less patient with him than I should have been. I just wanted to be with two little boys and suddenly to only have one. I mean I was in the depths of grief. I just kept saying why? Why can't I have two little children here? You're just so bitterly trying to fight this grief you just don't know what you're doing. At the same time he was going through a lot of health problems as well and you think how can all this happen? I've cried, and cried and cried and cried, I still do. Jacob says to me: 'Mummy where's your smile gone? ......
Briony, mother of baby boy Samuel (stillborn at forty-three weeks).

The previous account suggests that the impact of the death of a child created an emotional distancing from her surviving child as she was preoccupied by her own grief. In talking about her son's health problems there is a sense of being overwhelmed and emotionally exhausted to the extent that she is no longer able to manage a smile for her son who notices that it has disappeared. Living amidst the grief of his mother it is evident that the death impacts more widely in the family. Similarly Dyregrov (1991), described grief as a crisis which affects the whole family and its history since it impacts upon its current development and its redirection following the loss. In this research several parents reflected upon the difficulty they had in coping with their own grief, whilst trying to care for surviving children at home.

In direct contrast with the previous narrative, the following account shows a concern for and protectiveness over surviving children.

The account is framed by events surrounding the death of a thirteen day old baby girl who was born in hospital and brought home without any seeming complications. At eleven days of age, the baby became distressed and was taken by ambulance to hospital where she was admitted as an emergency. The surviving siblings were two (Daniel) and three years of age (Harry) at the time:

R: That's the thing they went to bed and we went away for two days and that's what he remembers. We followed the ambulance down Saturday morning, they [two sons] came down the Sunday. So from going to seeing their baby sister to like what they saw. Then they started crying. Harry is the angry one. If you think about it he was nineteenth months old, it was horrific. They can't control their feelings. When we got home, there were piles and piles of sympathy cards. He just put his arm out and swept the lot. We are trying to take away their bitterness, their grief, their loneliness. But since then Harry has never slept properly. It's like um if we go out we have to make sure, even now he wants to make sure we are coming home. We found that they have not really recovered from it, not properly...............

Christina, mother of baby girl Ella-Leina (born at forty weeks, lived for thirteen days).

The children described thus far, have not been interviewed directly so these are not their voices but that of their parents. It is outside the scope of this thesis to discuss children and their grief in great depth and one which is based upon their own perspective (see work on *'forgotten mourners'* by Hindmarch, 1995:37). Yet this narrative illuminates other complexities which may be present for men and women and their families. For example in the previous narrative, the respondent is grieving for the loss of her own daughter in addition to witnessing the emotional responses of her surviving children. Consequently, the space by which the mother is able to attend to her own emotional needs has to be negotiated to include all members of the family.

In contrast to the previous account, other respondents who have surviving children discuss some of the ways in which siblings offer sentiments which serve to ease the sense of desolation which can be felt by a death even several years later:

R: It's my son more than the others who remind me of him [baby who died]. Now and again he just comes out with something. Recently, he said 'do you know I wish I had a little brother, it's really sad I haven't got him isn't it, I would really like someone to play with'. I found out he was doing R.E (religious education), and they had to write about ten things they would pray to God for. The first one was 'that my brother Billy was alive'. That was the first on his list of prayers and I thought he's quite a sensitive little soul…………..

Susie, mother of baby boy Billy (born at thirty-eight weeks, lived for nine hours).

While the poignant words of an adolescent provided a source of comfort for a mother, the following narrative by a male respondent provided a source for coping:

R: Getting up in the morning was hard work. I didn't want to get up, life was pretty rubbish and I stayed in bed. Mille [daughter] was two and a half at the time and Selena [wife] got up before I did. She thought I ought to get up and do something, just go and see Millie, it made her feel better. I didn't realise at that point how useful Millie was going to be. Because of her we were able to...... she did so much for us we didn't realise it at all, she was a bright and bubbly two and a half year old. She wanted to do colouring and watch CBeebies [television programmes for children] and eat chocolate and just the normal things a two and a half year old wants to do, and you have to do those things as well. That part of life doesn't change and it can't change. So you have to get up out of bed and you have to do things for them. Two and half is a magical age and they are such wonderful people to have around, they do silly things and make you laugh. She was a good enough reason as any to want to get up out of bed in the morning to feed her and play with her and watch her do things. That's one of the biggest things I thought that helped us get through, certainly in the early days.................

Dan, father of baby boy, Jack (born at thirty-eight weeks, lived for two days).

What the previous narrative suggests is that the demands placed on caring for a young child affect the extent to which this father is able to be with his grief. There is a sense of personal identity which is maintained as a father to a boy who died and parenting a daughter who lives and who provides a purpose for living. The usual daily demands made by the surviving child have offered a potential anchor and a distraction from grief. For others, surviving children provide a way of publicly validating the grief of parents and of personifying the baby. This provides a source of comfort as the following account demonstrates in reference to the comments of a surviving child:

R: At her funeral, at Abbie's [baby who died] funeral she was the only child there. It went really quiet at one point.... and she's very articulate. She just pointed at Abbie's coffin and said to Tim [partner]: 'baby in there, baby in there'. She knew you know. When we go to the cemetery she kisses her fingers, and rubs her cross...........

Tina, Mother of baby girl Abbie (stillborn at forty weeks).

200

This account demonstrates how a parent is able to identify with the compassion and the energy of the living child, and who socially, legitimizes the death of the baby and grief of the mother. At the funeral, the baby who has died is identified, personified and validated as a person who existed. Further, the child who died is nurtured by her big sister at the graveside which represents a source of comfort for the mother.

What these accounts have shown is that respondents may be predisposed to behave in different ways to their surviving children and which for many do not represent emotionally distancing relationships. What they demonstrate is the difficulty in finding the resources to engage with daily life particularly when the losses are more recent. Further, these accounts show an extent of protectiveness which mirrors that of subsequent children described in Chapter 6, since the death forces parents to confront that which they were unable to control: the death of their child. As a bereaved parent they are dealing with the changes in how they see themselves and their connections to their deceased and surviving children.

The strength or weakness of a parent's connectedness with their children and with others (family and friends); and the extent to which they rely on these relationships to the maintenance of their identity, affects the resources they are able to draw upon.

Relationship with Family

Similar to the findings of other studies (Dent and Stewart, 2004; Lasker and Toedter, 1991; Riches and Dawson, 2000), the responses of relatives can mediate bereaved parents responses to loss. In particular, over half of the sample of twenty one women referred to their own mother as being supportive, whilst others described their mothers and mother–in-laws as being insensitive or unsupportive.

When women in this research described their own mothers as being supportive, this was in terms of emotional support. In the following example, the respondent was encouraged to re-engage with life by taking a trip to a local town:

R: I started to get like I wouldn't go out the flat or anything so it was like a month later Mum said right your Dad and I are going up to Barnstaple and we want you to get on the train and there's the money for your taxi down and back and we've paid for your ticket you meet us there…… just to get me to do it. I was doing really well and then it was the first of everything, and the first of everything is really hard and there was a new born baby there crying. Mum was total panic and like right we're gonna go to another café. I said, even though tears were streaming down my face, No Mum I've got to…. . Afterwards they got me that [shows me a teardrop of an Amber crystal necklace]. Yeah that's my teardrop of Amber for Rose [baby who died] which mum bought me and that is very special… because whenever I'm stressed I put the Amber on, I always put it on because it feels so close to her [baby who died]………..
Trudy, mother of baby girl Rose (stillborn at twenty-eight weeks).

Several women were able to recall similar types of support, though for others this was not forthcoming:

R: I have tried to discuss it [death of baby Lara] with my mother and she changes the subject every single time, she finds it very uncomfortable so I just stopped bringing it up. I would have thought that the one thing, the one person and the one place where I could get the most support and it ended being the least supportive. I found more support through SANDS and a company of strangers than I did from my own family………….
Claire, mother of baby girl Lara (stillborn at forty-one weeks).

202

It can be seen that the absence of a family history in which the baby is known can lead to assumptions that the loss was insignificant and could explain the grandmother's responses to loss. While the mother perceives the response as insensitive, it is an experience which is reflected in other respondent's accounts:

R: That is the worst thing you can do is not talk about it, just because we get upset that's not a bad thing. The worst thing is to ignore you, you've just lost a baby and you're treated like a leper because they are too embarrassed to be with you. Unfortunately my mother in law was quite unpleasant actually I have to say, quite unpleasant. She caused all sorts of problems with husband's sister about the way I was in it and what about her. She said: - "I was unhappy on the day of the funeral and nobody comforted me". I was thinking hang on a minute… this isn't about you. That was very difficult……….
Susie, mother of baby boy Billy (born at thirty-eight weeks, lived for nine hours).

These accounts of relationships with relatives have been selected since they represent some women's concern that their mother was insensitive. While it immediately appears that these relatives' responses are insensitive they reveal in themselves the consequences of loss for all family members. In the first account, the grandmother is 'too uncomfortable' which suggests that the loss grieves her also. Further, it can be seen that the death in the last account, has affected people more widely.

Ironically, it is precisely because this grandmother expressed her emotionality which led to the disintegration of the relationship in the first instance.

Indeed, while this was perceived as highly insensitive by the respondent, it nevertheless exposes the vulnerabilities in these encounters and the consequences of a mistimed expression. This sense of emotional distancing from relatives was a prominent theme which was repeated elsewhere:

R: Andy's [husband] Mum is very direct with her speech and If I say I am having a bad day she says you've just got to remember he's gone and I'm like yeah well I do know that….. he's dead. That is the reality of it but it doesn't seem real. It feels like someone is going to hand me my baby back and say sorry we're having a joke with you……
Angela, mother of baby boy Ollie (born at forty weeks, lived for twelve days).

Together these accounts of narratives with a mother-in-law are also characteristic of the way these families communicate which determines whether a bereaved parent's unique sense of loss is validated. Indeed, the extent to which members have established habits of listening to one another and their stories will influence the willingness of members to listen and to translate painful emotions into personal narratives and meaning. This suggests that some families are able to explore the meaning of the death whilst others, are reluctant to express their thoughts. Indeed families which accommodate differing views may be more open to accepting the range of emotions which accompany grief and, thus, be more open to negotiating new connections which accommodate the loss.

Generational differences may further explain grandparents' responses since they represent outdated ways of thinking about grief (Cecil, 1996). Consequently, several parents in this research remain disappointed by what they perceive to be inadequate support by their parents and mother-in laws. This demonstrates the way modern society lacks guidelines because there is no script as to how grandparents and others should respond to loss. Further, it is precisely because grandparents grieve that their capacity to support their bereaved children is diminished. Similarly, the responses of siblings demonstrate families varying ways of coping with loss:

R: When they [brother and sister] were actually up the crematorium they walked out, they said they couldn't cope with it and went to the... straight out to the pub where we were going afterwards... just walked straight out. I think how did they think we were coping then?............
Jim, father of baby girl Ella-Leina (born at forty weeks, lived for fourteen days).

This accounts contrasts significantly with the following narrative concerning a respondent's brother who is an uncle to the baby who died:

204

R: By the time he [brother] had arrived at the hospital I had already said goodbye to Ollie [baby who died] and he really wanted to see him, and said can I see him. So he went off with one of the nurses. My Mum was out getting me a glass of water or something and she saw this nurse rushing out in floods of tears, and she said that he [brother] had not only picked him up and held him and had a look at him, he sang/and talked to him. So it felt really, really special.... Yeah, like he would have done had he been alive almost. It really got to her, because he was only, only nineteen or something. So we asked 'L' [brother] if he would carry him to the grave since he had held him once before......

Wynnie, mother of baby boy Bryn (stillborn at forty weeks).

These narratives suggest that the differences in grieving among family members reflect the range of connections that existed prior to the death. The role of an uncle or aunt are defined and differentiated both by culture and by the working through of the family's own unique development (Nadeau, 1998).

Thus, each member of the family as the narratives suggest, is likely to have bonded with the child who has died according to the closeness both emotionally and chronologically to other siblings.

What is interesting about the previous account of sibling support is that it is unique to this research. It is an account which concerns a young man who is less habituated to conventions and norms. His actions are significant as they positively mediated the respondent's experience of loss by creating memories which helped with a sense of coping.

What remains from many accounts is the difficulty in finding empathic interlocutors. These seeming insensitivities of others I have argued, say more about grandparents' vulnerabilities and grief to reveal a death which has wider ramifications within the family. In others there is a degree of insensitivity which exposes the self to silences which respondents must learn to live with and which can amount to a debilitating social script. This is marked by respondents' reference to perceptions of insensitivity the consequences of which manifest in confusion, uncertainty and an emotional distancing in relationships.

Similarly, respondents' narratives suggest that the responses by friends and colleagues mediate parents' experiences of grief and loss. While it is not possible to consider these narrative parts in full within this chapter, they nevertheless serve to complement much of the varying responses to loss which are derived from familial networks. This seeming lottery of support resonates with respondents' accounts of their relationships with health professionals.

Relationships with Health Professionals

> *"The death of a child is one of the most devastating experiences that a parent can have and the quality of care at the end of life and after the child's death can have a major impact on the family's grieving."* (Royal College of Paediatrics and Child Health, 2004, quoted in Schott et al, 2007:145)

In Chapter 2 I argued that professional responses to perinatal loss vary significantly and in this study, even within the same hospital. While Leon (1992:366) reports that professional support in the perinatal loss encounter has improved, current practices are not optimal. He further argues that support tends to be institutionalised with professionals interacting with parents according to the detailed behavioural protocols rather than adopting an empathic awareness of the unique dimensions of perinatal loss.

In this research, the benefits of professional support vary among parents whose child is stillborn. Even in more positive accounts respondents note a lack of empathy and professional sensitivity. Several women complained about the midwife and doctors lack of interpersonal skills. The following accounts are from respondents, who owing to signs of distress from their baby, were waiting as emergency cases for ultrasound scans in hospital:

R: How to deal with it - it was just awful, it was like a carry on film. That is the only way I can describe it. This guy arrived and said: *"Oh I don't normally do ultrasound scans I'm not sure if I'm looking at the baby's heart or no*t." I'm thinking are you for real? Are you the person, the first person to arrive in this emergency and you do not know what you're doing? It was a reg (registrar) – I thought what are you doing here then? It makes you feel just really angry. I felt for a long time that I'd just been bloody raped. Just a piece of meat on a butcher's block oh well, this is an emergency who wants to do it then?
Paula, mother of baby girl Beth (born at forty weeks, lived for seventeen hours).

R: There were three of them that did it (health professionals). I think I knew deep down inside before I even got there that there were something way out, that there was something wrong. The first one that did it she was like messing about and trying to find a heartbeat. She was like I'll go and get somebody else I can't find it and this other one came in and she couldn't find anything either. They got the obstetrician in and he couldn't find one. I knew then that we lost her but then the next morning I thought everything would be fine....We came away like bizarre. You think that when you get past weeks. I never ever dreamt in a million years that I would get that far and something... I'd never heard of it before to be honest.... Came away, how do you tell people, they were like what? When we said we've lost 'N', they were like who? They thought I'd lost my grandma. It was like we'll just tell you your baby's died - come back in the morning. At the time I thought this is madness. I went back on the Tuesday morning and they did the scan and then they gave me a tablet [to induce the birth]......
Sandie, mother of baby girl Katie (stillborn, thirty-six weeks).

The first account demonstrates a situation made worse by the manner in which it is addressed, which has consequences since it continues to anger the respondent several years after the death of her child.

The situation described in the second account, lends itself to a sense of the surreal such as that referred to by Layne as scientific dis-synchronicity. In writing about miscarriage, Layne's (2003:86) reference to this dis-synchronicity refers to learning about the death and then giving birth to a dead baby. In between, the woman is physically and visibly still pregnant, yet has to walk around with the knowledge that she is carrying a dead baby inside of her. This sense of dis – synchronicity is demonstrated in the previous account as the respondent refers to a sort of madness as she tries to comprehend what has happened.

This particular narrative has been selected since it reflects respondents' experiences of professional support more widely during interviews. In particular, the stillbirth narratives reflect to a greater extent, a tendency for more negative references to professional care during labour:

R: They kept asking us what we were going to do with the body? They were asking us about twenty times while I was in labour. We had already made the decision and already told them we wanted a private burial and funeral rather than let the hospital arrange it. They kept asking and asking and asking, and it was 'we have already told you. I don't want to talk about that right now anyway'. There were lots of things like that..........
Carla, mother of baby girl Leia (stillborn, twenty-four weeks).

Following the birth:
R: I wish a really kind midwife had come in and said your baby is really beautiful, just someone to be compassionate towards her and to have treated her as a human being instead of as hospital waste. When she was born they carried her out in one of those cardboard trays and that really got to me because that is what they put the rubbish in. They didn't at any point refer to her like she had been a human being. She was though and she was our daughter and our baby and what we hoped would be a life and there was no acknowledgement of that.............

The previous example demonstrates quite clearly the perceived lack of empathy afforded the respondent who would have needed very sensitive support at such a critical time as the labour knowing that when her baby was born, she would be dead, and then, to her dismay, be carried out as hospital waste. It is difficult for the mother to discern let alone comprehend the reason for the approach adopted by a professional in this situation. Mahan and Calica (1997) attempt to explain when they argue that while professionals use their own unique emotional responses to help in their work with bereaved parents, repeated exposure to loss leads some professionals to desensitise as a defence mechanism against professional 'burnout'. This is discussed more widely in Chapter 3, and in part may explain why even within the same hospital and on the same maternity ward, parents experienced differences in the attitudes of staff to their needs:

R: Somehow she just knew what to say, what to do. She even brought in things for Jacob [first son]. It's just sweet little gestures. I will never ever, ever forget her kindness. Another day, another midwife came in and she just didn't have that nature. It's just your character…………..

Briony, mother of baby boy Samuel (stillborn at forty-three weeks).

R: With the midwife she was the morning staff and very bustly. I was just an ordinary patient on an ordinary ward. When she brought Abbie [baby who died] in to me in this Moses basket there wasn't even any compassion shown to 'R', there wasn't any comment made. The midwife the previous night treated her like you know a live baby, she took a photograph of her, she wrapped her up, she looked into her face. She didn't sort of think oh this baby's gone you know. She even made the comment that even out of stillborn babies that she has delivered that Abbie had a very pretty and peaceful face…..

Tina, mother of baby girl Abbie (stillborn at forty weeks).

The sense of confusion described in previous narratives exposes encounters which are in part, emotionally distancing. For example, the professional obsession with a babies bodies and what are regarded as their mortal remains reduces their personification to that of waste products to be disposed of in cartons usually used for urine, sick and excrement. Moreover respondents' accounts reveal that their role as grieving men and women is limiting, since they have been both institutionally and professionally steered towards certain narratives which are about processes. These particular barriers to emotionality overshadow these more positive and sensitive encounters. The consequences of this are that these bereavement narratives remain unheard, they are left to fester in anger, in shame, and in frustration.

These encounters contrast with the majority of respondents' neonatal death experiences which feature professionals who 'act' in empathic ways, thereby supporting respondents' emotional welfare in addition to acknowledging the magnitude of their loss. This raises questions more widely as to the extent to which loss and bereavement is viewed as a core part of midwives training.

While it is not within the remit of this thesis to interview midwives and explore their attitudes and perceptions of the care they provide, what these examples highlight are the differences in the support received across British maternity hospitals.

In this third reading about relationships with health professionals, I explore respondents' experiences on the neonatal ward since they represent more empathic dialogic exchanges and practices. It can be seen then, that the role of nursing staff is critical in acknowledging the impact of the loss. This extends to practices which enable men and women to have loving memories of their child:

R: It was lovely up there [bereavement suite]. I bathed him and dressed him. It sounds really odd but it was the loveliest thing to be able to do to give him a bath and to get him dressed as you would any other baby. There are some nice memories from that point of view. My abiding memory was the time I spent with him, which was a lovely time, well as lovely as it can be.............
Susie, mother of baby boy Billy (born at thirty-eight weeks, lived for nine hours).

What is poignant about this account is that it brings into awareness comparisons with the stillbirth narratives. The extent to which respondents of stillborn children were either offered or encouraged in these practices varied significantly. Some respondents were asked if they wanted to bathe their baby, whilst others were not irrespective of their gestational age of the child.

These comparisons are made since respondents later learn from others what they could have had, which is a few more moments with their child. This later knowing causes regret and guilt as respondents feel they should have known and should have asked for these special moments, yet felt 'swept along by a system'. Yet these memorialising practices facilitate parenting and the creation of memories which the respondent can refer to positively.

For this reason the following narrative has been selected since it represents other more subtle yet compassionate ways to support parents on the neonatal ward:

R: It was Angela's [wife] birthday and on the Sunday it was Father's day. That Neonatal unit I can't fault them. On that Father's Day when I went in there was even a bar of chocolate to Daddy from Ollie [baby who later died]. It was little things like that, that shows that they .... Even the nurses there said this isn't like - this isn't another baby that comes and goes - it affects us. I think it did affect them as well, especially a term baby. To see a full term baby die like that, that is not an everyday occurrence is it?
Andy, father of baby boy Ollie (born at forty weeks, lived for twelve days).

This account lends particular insight to professional responses to loss. Of note is the sense of meaning attached to a child since his death is felt more widely and has touched professionals. This dialogic exchange between a respondent and health professional is crucial since the respondent is acknowledged as a father to this child, a status which he is unable to claim more socially when he leaves the hospital without his son. This account has also shown a sense of professional vulnerability which reveals the enormity and difficulty some nurses have in conducting work in the neonatal unit. These tasks are social, emotional as well as medical and employed in varying situations. For example, the following account describes professional approaches around a baby's dying moments which represented the first time the respondent had held her baby following his care in an incubator:

R: He died with just the two of us. Um, and we had this sort of you hold, him, you hold him. He was obviously dying as there was a great gasping for breath. This junior doctor and a nurse kept popping in and we had some wonderful nurses and they were so special. In the end I think he died in my arms which is in that photo [points to mantelpiece] because the doctor came in and said yes, he pronounced him dead and he had to sign a time.......
Mary, mother of baby boy Christopher (born at forty weeks, lived for four days).

These professional practices demonstrate respect for these memorable moments with a child.

These are events which the respondent is able to consider with a poignant yet positive regard for professionals a theme which she maintained throughout the interview. Similarly, the following account has been selected since it represents practices which most respondents of neonatal death experiences represent. It concerns a child's withdrawal from life support and their dying moments:

R: We wanted to go outside when they did it and they were great and they put him in a little pram. We went and sat down on a bench and one nurse came with us. She was really good. She took all these tubes out and for a few moments... and he died in our arms. You know of all the ways he could go, that was as good as it could get really. We spent at least an hour in the wooded area of the hospital and just sat in the woods with him and the nurse she just wandered off and was keeping an eye on us in the distance and let us get on with it. That was nice, it was the first time we'd seen him and held him without a load of tubes and all the ventilator and all that. He just looked like an ordinary baby and he looked like he was asleep.... ...

Andy, father of baby boy Ollie (born at forty weeks, lived for twelve days).

These accounts demonstrate how institutional medical procedures (pronouncing death and time of death, withdrawal from life support) are inextricably linked to emotional management in that they are embedded in the actions and language of these particular professionals. These interactions can be seen as rituals and exchanges which mobilise empathic practices. They acknowledge the enormity of the loss and affirm the status of mother and father. These practices are comparable to respondents' narratives of stillborn children, which are in keeping with the findings of Lovell's (1983) stillbirth research in London hospitals.

It is suggested that these varying approaches come about for several reasons and in part relate to the discussion in chapter three about 'emotion work' and 'status shields'. This is considered in the context of Freund's (1990) understanding of power domination and social control.

As Freund himself explains: *"External social structural factors such as one's position in different systems of hierarchy or various forms of social control can influence the conditions of our existence, how we respond and apprehend these conditions and our sense of embodied self."* (1990:461)

This embodied form of emotion, and professional activity in a socio-cultural context are inextricably linked. As can be seen in these accounts emotional modes of being can be positive or deeply unpleasant, the crucial difference being that they represent being empowered or disempowered. This is linked to the conditions of men's and women's existence throughout these particular narrations. These varying accounts reflect men's and women's social position and status in hospital, revealing the resources men and women have to define the self as mother or father and to counter the invalidation by such significantly powerful professionals. To this end, those who occupy the least powerful positions in the social hierarchy are at greater risk of being invalidated, of feeling powerless and angered by these distressing embodied experiences. As Freund further explains: (1990): *"One's positions and the roles that accompany them in various systems of social hierarchy shape the conditions in which one lives. This position influences access to resources. It may also determine the forms of emotional – social control to which one is subject as well as the severity of the impact of these controls have on the person. Such a process may mean internalising the emotional definitions that others impose on what we are and should be."* (1990:470)

It can be seen that if stillbirth represents an invalidation of motherhood, and, thus, occupation of a lower social status. This compares to women's counterparts on the neonatal unit. It is with embodied feelings of powerlessness that respondents refer to organisations such as SANDS for emotional assistance.

213

Support Groups

> *"One kind of death is no less awful than another. All deaths lead to stress pain and change in almost every aspect of a family's life. Regardless of the way their children die, parents speak in the same language. In each instance, the disarray may take its own shape, but is always there."* **Silverman (2000: 132)**

In the last twenty years voluntary organisations such as SANDS have developed support groups across the UK and have extended their activities into New Zealand and Australia. Similarly, Layne (2003) notes that this trend has occurred in the United States with over five hundred 'SHARE' (Source of Help in Arising and Resolving Experiences) groups. These developments argue Layne (2003:69), are in response to the cultural denial of perinatal loss and are a means of defining the death of a baby as a legitimate source of grief. In this research, one of the most commonly cited reasons for attending a support group was because of complaints about the perceived insensitivities of others. The following accounts have been selected since they represent some of the reasons why men in this research have found such support in this way useful:

R: I had the courage to go to the group but it was very hard to step out and make your grief public and very, very difficult.....It's almost like a secret club that people you know have been through it because you don't ram it down your friends' throat or go up to strangers and talk about it, it's very strange.....

Ian, father of baby girls Melody and Joy (born at twenty-seven weeks, lived for two hours).

R: I was hugely trepidatious about it, I kind of though uugh. I couldn't think of anything worse than going to talk about it with loads of other people so I was very scared about going but we did and um, yeah...I don't really like speaking in groups but I found that space incredibly useful to do. Just to, to be able to just open up a set of questions and then obviously to hear other people's stories was important as well. I don't really know why that is, but it does seem to be incredibly useful. Just that kind of sharing that seems alien to everyday life. I find that kind of 'family of people', that group kind of just knows where you've been, you know. There is something really important about that....

Karl, father of baby boy Bryn (stillborn at forty weeks).

The purpose for meeting is to break the silence around a very difficult issue. Indeed, while reference to talking about this with friends concerns a self imposed silence, these accounts also expose the lack of a cultural script in which these voices can be heard more readily. As has been shown elsewhere in this thesis, such topics represent that which is difficult to listen to and contemplate: the death of a child. It is this and others responses to the loss which inform respondents' attendance at these meetings. In this research, women have attended these groups for similar reasons to that of men:

R: Suddenly you discover so many people who have been through it but we don't speak out, it's this terribly British thing where you don't' show your grief. I think that's one of the worst things that were expected to get over things, we're expected to cope and not show our grief and as a result quite a few of the... You don't have any support other than that organised by other sufferers like the SANDS groups and things.....
Ruth, mother of baby girls Melody and Joy (born at twenty-seven weeks, lived for two hours).

R: For most of the time [everyday life] I feel like I'm putting on an act all the time because people don't want you to talk about it. If you're having a really bad day and the phone rings you answer and say Hi really chirpy. It's only when you go to the group you feel normal and you can say I am still thinking about her and I do want to talk about her and I am missing her you know. Its kind of nice to be able to do that because even with my closest friends even if I mention it they kind of get all awkward and they don't know what to say and they don't what to do. I think well you've got no idea and then I think well no they haven't......
Christina mother of baby girl Ella-Leina (born at forty weeks and lived for thirteen days).

These accounts reflect for these respondents, a broader social and cultural landscape in which discussions about loss are confined to a sub-culture of bereaved parents. Several of these women have been active in public campaigns loss in Westminster (March, 2009) and some have published accounts of their loss to raise awareness of these issues which are so pertinent to them. For other respondents fund raising and enacting change through liaison with maternity committees gives purpose to and meaning for their present lives.

While the accepted wisdom is that attendance to a group is typically a westernised and white, middle-class phenomenon, several respondents were in receipt of social assistance in the form of means tested benefits and social housing and were actively engaged in developing and facilitating groups. Writers such as Layne (2003) and McCleod, (2008) suggest that the proliferation of baby loss organisations and hospital bereavement services reflect the cultural acceptance of talking in a therapeutic setting. Further, academic and popular press have made this form of loss more visible. Yet members of support groups attest that a culture of silence around this subject still permeates (Layne, 2003: 68). This is reflected by several respondents' narratives and suggests that despite the activity and discussion about baby loss there is consistent silence surrounding the actual experience in wider society (Simmonds and Rothman, 1992:2).

Thus, it cannot be assumed that voluntary organisations such as SANDS can meet the need of every individual parent whose baby has died. While the exception, there were two respondents who had tried on several occasions to get help but their phone calls were never returned and as a consequence they had to pay for therapeutic services elsewhere. This also suggests that voluntary organisations are limited in their resources, which needs to be borne out in the development of bereavement support in the community, following the parents' departure from hospital.

Conclusion

To conclude, this reading has been concerned with men and women's relationships with their partners and significant others (surviving children, family, friends, work colleagues, health professionals) and support groups. It has been suggested that many men and women feel isolated and angered following their loss, which they attribute to other people's lack of acknowledgement. While several respondents appreciated the emotional support of partners, others were more critical owing to subjective perceptions, to which the traditional gendered emotional response debate proffered little understanding.

It was argued that this represented a wider cultural misunderstanding of masculinity and bereavement such that a more useful interpretation could be framed within a sociological understanding of men's and women's grief. To this end, it was suggested that unlike the parenting of live children, relationships between bereaved men and women lacked representation both culturally and socially.

An emphasis upon relationships exposed the complex nature of such interactions with relatives, in particular with mother-in-laws who it was argued, represented the generational differences inherent in these relationships. These relationships appeared superficial representing as they did an emotional distancing similar to that displayed by some health professionals.

It was suggested that men and women were bombarded with so many competing perspectives (relatives, professionals and their own) that they struggled to hold onto one recognisable as their own. In this saturation of stories with varying points of view, respondents almost become 'written on' from the outside. This could be found in the dialogic exchange with health professionals in the stillbirth narratives when compared with those of the neonatal deaths.

These accounts exposed a social hierarchy employed by professionals which conferred a status that demoted men's and women's personhood to non-parent. It was this lack of deference to parents' whose child was stillborn which had consequences for their sense of self and ambivalent role.

In these twenty-seven accounts of stillbirth and neonatal death many of the men and women interviewed, argued that the responses of others (partners, children, family members, and professionals) mediated their own embodied responses to their experience of loss. I have suggested that these responses are consequential since men and women in this research continue to experience their sense of self as neither non-parent or parent but more as a misfit. Where the responses of others were perceived as positive this facilitated a sense of coping; compared to negative experiences which compounded feelings of neglect and of a sense of not belonging.

Following from the previous readings about respondents' accounts of their relationships with others, the next reading will be concerned with the social and cultural discourses in society; such as beliefs, parenting and continuing bonds with the child who has died.

CHAPTER 8. Placing People Within Cultural Contexts and Social Structures

Introduction

Chapter 7 explored how social relationships affect the way bereaved parents make sense of the death of their baby and how friends, family, colleagues and health professionals helped or hindered adjustment to bereavement. Following Mauthner and Doucet's (1998:132) voice centred relational method this chapter explores the ways in which the broader social, political and cultural contexts surrounding bereavement can lead to varying interpretations of the death of a baby and to differing grief reactions. I argue that some of the problems bereaved parents face arises from the dissonance between mainstream culture and the culture of bereavement. The consequences of the differences between these two cultures are the lack of sensitivity, avoidance and impatience with bereaved parents' perceived preoccupation with the death of their baby.

Traditionally, models of grief suggest that following a period of mourning, the bereaved should sever their ties to the deceased. It will be shown in this fourth and final reading that men and women do not want to forget the child who has died; rather they want to continue a bond which provides emotional solace. I provide evidence to support these claims through the representational systems men and women employ to retain a sense of the child in their lives. A case is made that these representations in the form of photographs and artefacts are a way of defining the baby as a real person. This is considered in light of the workplace which provides either opportunities for coping with grief or represents a limiting approach to supporting the bereaved in their work.

It will be shown that the work place acts as a refuge for the few, yet as a place to be avoided for those whose whole career trajectory is disrupted by practices and colleagues responses to the death. This sense of disruption is extended to a professional discourse due in part to institutional procedures and varying approaches to loss and location of care.

219

It is these practices which reflect cultural norms and social values more widely in relation to stillbirth and neonatal death. To this end, I conclude by arguing that an exploration of the social structures and cultural contexts of men's and women's experiences exposes that which is a social problem, a lack of a coherent script by which to respond to the bereaved in the modern age.

Continuing Bonds with the Baby

The concept of continuing bonds has been well documented over the last sixty years in the medical, psychological and counselling literature (see more recent work, Bennett and Bennett, 2000; Dyregrov, 2008; Silverman, 1996) and has emerged as a strong theme within this study. It is argued that the sense of presence of the baby in a parent's life does not occur at a single and early stage of bereavement as suggested by the literature, but can last a lifetime. The view that dominates scientific discourse is that the experience of the relationship with the child is illusory and a symptom of a broken heart and a mind in chaos, or otherwise a longing and a search for the person who has died (Bennett, and Bennett, 2000:139).

Indeed, Western theories of bereavement stress that successful resolution from grief occurs when the bereaved person severs their emotional ties to the deceased (Marwitt and Klass, 1996: 297). What is questioned here is that in the context of the death of a baby, when does a parent stop being a parent to the child who has died?

Following Bennett and Bennett's (2000:139) empirical study of accounts of the deceased as a feature in the survivor's life, an alternative interpretation is presented within the discussion of respondents' continuing bond with their deceased child. This enables the bond to be viewed as 'real' and 'natural' and evidence of the continued link between the parent and their baby. It is suggested, that both these discourses are cultural artefacts which are rational and traditional. In a search to find meaning to their experiences both these discourses are accessed by parents.

In parents' narratives the death does not seem able to sever the bond once shared with their child, and, thus, grief can be viewed as a transition from loving in presence to loving in absence. The majority of respondents provided examples of a continuing relationship with their baby who had died. In searching for an understanding of their experience however, many parents became isolated:

R: I did go out a lot even though some of the time I went out and just drove to go somewhere. Occasionally I took 'J' [first son] to the child minders. I never used to come back here [home] I used to go off and remember driving and with this music from his musical toy [the baby's toy] and I'd just cry and cry and cry and sometimes ... I got into the routine from the time that Christopher [baby who died] was buried. I used to go up to the grave every single day and the first time I didn't.. when we went away..... it was almost painful. I felt disloyal to him.............

Mary, mother of baby boy Christopher (born at forty-two weeks, lived for four days).

The previous narrative describes a mother's experience in the first year following the death of her son. Her account is discussed in relation to the representation of the child to herself and how this interacts with her daily life. There is a sense of disequilibrium and dissociation with general life as she travels alone listening to her baby's music.

It is a reality which she describes as routine as she tries to find a way of continuing the bond with her baby by visiting his grave everyday. While this describes the respondent's experiences in the first year of her bereavement, the bond is continued in other ways over the mother's life course. In the interview she often referred to her baby's photograph which has its place on the mantelpiece alongside her other children.

As this narrative and others given by parents in this study suggest, the death of a child can have an effect on a parent's ability to find credible meaning to their experience and reconcile it with previous assumptions about the life they lived prior to the death (Riches and Dawson, 2000: 103).

221

Indeed, in previous chapters respondents have spoken about the way life becomes surreal and that there was dissociation from people they would usually have relationships with. This is in keeping with the findings of Klass's (1996:199) longitudinal ethnographic study of bereaved parents. He states that when a child dies parents perceive that their lives have stopped while other people's go on. In this study several respondents spoke about their experiences of trying to understand other people's responses to their loss. Yet other responses served to reaffirm a continuing bond in the following account:

R: I remember someone saying to me once, would you rather it never happened, wouldn't it be better if that year you were pregnant with Jo [baby who died], and lost him, none of that had happened? I can remember saying to them well no because I feel the joy of having had him outweighs the loss of having lost him. I've got something a lot of people haven't got. I've got a child in heaven who is in my heart all the time and who I love as much as I love Thomas [living child], and wouldn't ever want that taken away................
Anna, mother of baby boy Thomas (stillborn, twenty-four weeks).

As a mother of a son who died in stillbirth she is aware that there is little in the way of the potential for an external dialogue with others by which to construct a memory and find meaning, as her son was seen by very few people. This is despite the bereavement literature's assertion that successful resolution to grief comes about through the provision of social support to the grieving person. The previous narrative demonstrates that the mother does not seek out the support of friends to provide meaning to her loss, rather she engages in a social process by which she re negotiates who her son was, what he meant to her and what he represents to her in her everyday life. On one level, this may reflect a personal faith in a place such as heaven, in which the child can be pictured or construed as being safe. On another, her focus upon her changed self suggests her son was and continues to be an abstract presence in her life. In finding meaning about the death, she reveals what she has become as an individual, which is a much more compassionate woman.

Similarly, Riches and Dawson's (2000:123) research findings from bereaved women suggest that mothers viewed significant change in themselves such as a new inner strength they found alongside the continuing pain of loss and an ongoing relationship with the child who died.

The majority of babies continued to exist as a presence in respondents' lives and in the conversations of parents. In various ways, respondents have described having an inner dialogue with their baby in the car, or at home and bringing them up to date with recent familial developments. Other men and women felt that they were being watched over and taken care of by their baby 'from the other side'. This theme featured strongly with parents who had visited psychic mediums (person who claims to be able to contact the dead) as a means of emotional solace, wanting the reassurance that their child continued to exist *somewhere*.

Similarly, the parents and adolescents from Klass (1996:199) and Hogan De Santis's (1992:159) study believed they would see the deceased child again when they died. This contrasts markedly from Bowlby's (1980) thesis concerning detachment and the severing of ties to the deceased, a model often cited as an important way to grieve (see Chapter 1). Yet, what this research and others such as Klass et al's have shown suggests that grief is about the transformation of the physical presence of the child into an abstract one, which far from being given up is something which is held onto.

Indeed, for several respondents, some of the other ways of retaining a continued presence of the deceased baby in their lives and within the family was through items associated with the child. For example, one respondent spoke about the baby's scent from the blanket she was wrapped in when taken out of the incubator. Another mother presented a crystal at the interview which was worn during the labour and which sits next to the photograph of the baby who died. All of these precious items serve to memorialise, personify and, thus, create a place for the baby in the parent's life.

These findings concur with Layne's (2003:112), study in which parents' narratives on pregnancy loss serves as a testament as to the importance of items. In one account, a baby's toy bear from the pre-planned nursery signifies to the parent that her child was 'a real baby with real baby things' (Layne, 2003: 113).

For most parents, a photograph of the baby signified the presence of the baby in the family. These precious photos adorned the central mantelpiece, wall or special place which could be viewed by visitors to parents' homes. Other respondents (though few), chose other 'special places' and disclosed that the picture of their baby was next to their side of the bed. This suggests that one way in which parents renegotiate the self following loss is how they demonstrate the baby's presence in the family to the outside world.

For some respondents the existence of the baby was to be reaffirmed by the acknowledgement of subsequent children in the family. The following account is by a mother who is aware she is expecting a baby girl at twenty-four weeks gestation following the death of her first baby daughter Elen eighteen months previously:

R: I've said to my friends that this baby is going to grow up knowing that she's had a sister and that while she's little maybe she'll come to the cemetery because I can't leave her at home. Equally when she's fifteen years old and she understands and she doesn't want to come I'm not going to drag her and make her. When she's growing up I'll point to her picture and say that's your sister Elen... ... .

Sophia, mother of baby girl Elen (born at twenty four weeks, lived for two hours).

The picture of the baby and the grave site are critical pieces of evidence that the baby existed. The continuing bond to the baby and her continued presence within the family is reliant upon the next child appreciating that her sister did exist. Part of the mother's wishes for her next daughter to appreciate the bond she has with the child who has died can be explored in the context of her grief.

For example, Klass (1996:201) suggests that the dynamics by which grief is resolved by parents involves a transformation of the inner representation of their child to the parents' social world. When the child's death is acknowledged and a continuing bond with the child is a socially shared reality, then the representation of the child to the parent is secure.

In the previous narrative the successful resolution to grief is not about the severing of the bond but integrating the child into the parent's life and into their social world. What this demonstrates is that parents reweave the lasting love with their deceased child into the larger, richly complex fabric of their lives (Attig, 2001: 34).

While many respondents found similar ways to integrate the deceased child into their life, the following narrative reveals the struggle some respondents face in trying to find ways to parent in their ambivalent status as a parent of a dead child, Jack:

R: There were things like designing a headstone to go on his grave and things like that. That was hard and put a lump in my throat designing a headstone for my son. That didn't' feel anything like right. It was the best we could have done for Jack and we always try and make sure Jacks' grave is always tended nicely and kept clean and that the flowers look nice. There are no nappies to change. There is nothing we can do for Jack practically, he is always in our minds and in our hearts, he is with us everywhere we go but there is nothing we can do for him……………
Dan father of baby boy Jack (born at forty weeks, lived for two days).

This account demonstrates that in trying to come to terms with the ambivalent bond with his baby, the father in the first instance separates his son from his sense of self. He talks about being unable to physically care for his child yet his son has been transformed into the father's inner world in his mind, in his emotional self and in his daily life.

For other respondents, a bond is strengthened by integrating the baby into the family on anniversaries. For example, for one mother, each anniversary of the birth and later death (following day) of her baby is marked by the whole family who each year take a trip to the theatre or to see a special sight in the British capital such as the 'London Eye'. The mother collects a souvenir to mark the day and places the special item in the baby's memory box (box of items which memorialise the baby for example photos and clothing). The following day, flowers are taken to the baby's grave to mark his anniversary.

As this mother explains:

R: The kids really enjoy it. In fact we even had a party one year I know it sounds strange we were up at my sister in law, the one I get on with really well with and she said: 'what do you want to do for his birthday' I had no idea. She said: 'we could have a party.' So we had a kid's birthday party. We had party hats, we had a cake, we had the whole lot, the whole nine yards. It was absolutely brilliant we had such a good day, the kids had a great time and it was all in his memory and that was about three years ago when he would have been about ten, so it would have been what you would do for a child at that age anyway. For the kids it's completely natural to do that. It keeps his memory alive with the children as well because they didn't know him. It's nice for me that we can be open about it……………
Susie, mother of baby boy Billy (born at thirty-nine weeks, lived for nine hours).

While it is not possible to obtain the surviving children's perspective and whether they shared their mother's sense of the baby in their lives, the anniversary of the baby's birthday represents the mother's continuing bond with her deceased child. The act of marking the day as a family in her son's memory involves her sister-in-law and suggests that the abstract presence of the child has extended into the mother's social network.

As respondents find a different equilibrium in their lives and new ways of understanding the world, so they find different ways in which to hold their child within the family. While the narratives suggest that this is on the whole accepted, of equal significance is how the death of a baby affects a parent's working life.

Parents' Work and Employment

The subject of employment was raised by several respondents when they spoke about the way the death of their baby had changed their perception of work. For several men and women, work proved difficult to return to and prompted a change in career. For example, one mother was employed in a senior position prior to the death of her baby and chose to undertake Saturday morning work as a shop assistant. Several respondents discussed their resumption of work and how this affected them. The following narrative describes both the difficulty and benefits of returning to her employment as a palliative care nurse:

R: Patients were really understanding and sent cards. I got some flowers and a card from work. Some people came up and asked how we were doing and said I'm really sorry. Other people didn't say anything at all, they didn't acknowledge it, and they didn't say anything. Two people that I work with, one of them I work with were brilliant and understanding. The other one, I'd never met before but he couldn't understand all this fuss and palaver over grief for a baby. He said it wasn't like she was fifteen and I'd had fifteen years of life with her to get to know her. He couldn't understand that the minute you find out you're pregnant you start the bond and I'd already bonded with her then... He saw it more like I was grieving for the lifestyle I'd lost of being a mother than the baby that I'd lost. His attitude was you're a year down the line now, you know, you should have got over it by now, how can you have all this grief and this problem over a baby that was only here for two hours, and I'm sure it's your lifestyle you're grieving over now. That's really difficult that, cos I made a conscious effort of not bringing my problems to work cos I used work as a bit of a scape goat. I actually could have a break for the eight and a half hours that I was at work. So I made a conscious effort not to bring the two together...............
Sophia, mother of baby girl Elen (born at twenty-four weeks, lived for two hours).

227

While insensitively placed, the remarks of a colleague exposes the difficulty the mother has at work while grieving for the death of her daughter as well as a loss of possibility of her social role as a mother. This lack of empathy was consequential for the respondent.

Sophia described in the interview how his attitude made her question her ability to carry out her work. She spoke about feeling under a great deal of pressure to prove she could do her work well and became extremely fearful that she would fail. She felt she had no option but to reduce her working hours and decline any new patients onto her case load. This account demonstrates the varying responses which have been talked about more widely in this thesis and which reflects the lack of cultural script available about the death of babies. While there are instances of empathy, in other cases there are none. In the previous account there is a lack of empathy and impatience by a colleague. It could be argued that the colleague, a nurse, responded according to the professional (defined by medicine) discourse to which he had become accustomed.

Having met with similar responses, other women stopped working in paid positions and undertook unpaid, volunteer work to raise funds for memorial gardens and for SANDS. There was the sense that the emotional pain of loss had to count for something and these activities were a way of finding meaning. For example, one respondent made clothes for premature babies for the hospital where her son died as a way of remaining close to him. Another respondent found a way to continue a bond to her baby by changing her job so she could work in the human resources department in the hospital where her baby had died. Both women described how this brought them solace. It could be argued that these accounts demonstrate that the meaning of the relationship and the significance of the parent-child bond contributes to the wrenching life readjustment that is required following loss.

Yet the depth and richness of the parent-child attachment bond and the way this is transformed following loss is largely ignored in the conceptual frameworks in the bereavement and psychiatric literature (Rubin, 1984:217). Rather attention is given to the degree of functionality at work at the expense of how the baby is remembered and recollected (Schechter and Rubin, 1994). Further, within the psychiatric literature there is little clarity on what is the most important issue when addressing the loss of a loved one. Rather, the focus upon function and dysfunction in the assessment of reactions to loss has largely overshadowed the independent feature of grief, particularly in relation to perinatal loss. Where it is mentioned, it is done sparingly (Leon, 1992).

This is despite recent legislation aimed at improving the rights of parents at work (Employment Act, 2002) and in particular fathers' paternity leave. Yet none of the respondents mentioned structural work practices in relation to having a baby and experiencing their death. As the narrative presented in this section suggests, it was the respondent's own initiative and decision to reduce her working hours, and not a policy which was presented by her employers. None of the other respondents mentioned any policy or management involvement in returning to work, and some of the ways this could be handled. Where some respondents discussed being unable to resume employment, for others, work served as a place by which to avoid their grief. Of these men and women, the majority continued in their occupation due to economic necessity and not choice.

Other than Riches and Dawson (1997, 2000) research on parents' grief following the death of a child, there is a dearth of research pertaining to bereavement and employment. Yet the accounts of employment given by respondents suggest that bereavement experiences can be mediated by factors such as whether or not the workforce and the workplace is sympathetic and knowledgeable about the impact of perinatal death. Where it is lacking then it could be argued that attitudes and values need to change to reflect more humane approaches to loss

229

Social Discourse, Expectations and Beliefs

Riches and Dawson (2000:50) argue that cultural beliefs and social conventions prompt some of the ways by which people express and control their feelings around the death of a loved one. This suggests that the significance of a death of a baby to society varies from culture to culture. While it is outside the remit of this thesis to consider cross national variances it is important to note that western societies comprise a cultural diversity of racial mixes and ethnic groups and belief systems. Further, the shifting boundaries of class, gender, age, nationality and community suggest that there is a lack of uniformity to the way the death of a baby in hospital is experienced, grieved for and supported (Parkes et al, 1997). This suggests that attitudes towards infant death in western modern society remain ambivalent and contradictory. This ambivalence towards other people's loss can be seen to extend into everyday social reality for men and women in this research. For example, one respondent describes reserving the right to receive free dental treatment following the stillbirth of her daughter (treatment which is provided free of charge for up to one year for mothers who have had a baby). Yet this was a right that the mother had to fight for at a time when she experienced a great sense of loss:

R: I had a stand up row at the dentist. I went up after my treatment and they charged me and I said, I'm entitled to this for nothing and she said no you've got to pay, and I said, no I don't. She [receptionist] rang up the dentist; he wouldn't come down and he said she has to pay. I said no I don't it's not my fault my baby died at birth. I walked out without paying and said right I tell you what I am going to do now, I'm going to the Citizens Advice Bureau and I'm going to find out and then I'm going to come back and tell you. I told my husband and he said: 'right I'm going to talk to them about this.' So he went up to see the dentist and he said: 'I want a guarantee that you will not do this to anybody again.' The dentist said: 'I can't guarantee that.' I just thought what a bastard; they're all money sucking greedy bastards!................
Lou, mother of baby girl Marie-Rose (stillborn at twenty-seven weeks).

While this demonstrates the perceived lack of sensitivity on the part of the dentist to the trauma faced by the mother, of note is the dentist's refusal to deal with the mother directly.

There is no acknowledgement for the grief experienced by the mother or apology for the challenge that she faced. This form of response was reflected in other parent's narratives and at times when the need for sensitivity could not have been greater.

In another account, both a mother and a father of baby 'A', describe the insensitivity and indifference of crematorium staff at the internment of the baby's ashes:

R: My Mum and Dad were late because of the Christmas traffic and this guy (at the crematorium) said: 'we'll have to start it if they're late.' He stuck a piece of paper to the side (box of ashes). It's an emotional day and the death of a baby……. and he marches across and we had two little boys in a pushchair, and he marches straight across all the headstones. It was awful…… We got to the grave and I looked in and there was this hole and they just tipped her in. I thought she was going to be put in a casket or a pot. I was just horrified. I think we were both just so shocked that we didn't say anything and um… he said flippantly: 'oh do what you want.' I was worried the wind took some of her ashes and she wouldn't be whole I know that sounds stupid doesn't it?
Christina, mother of baby girl Ella-Leina (born at thirty-nine weeks, lived for thirteen days).

Following further incidences (one in which a small bear bought by the baby's brothers had been removed by cemetery staff and placed elsewhere), the parents applied to the Home Office to have their baby's ashes buried elsewhere. The event was clearly handled with a significant lack of sensitivity and by a member of staff whose attitude was indifferent towards the baby, the parents and family members. This is, however, the exception to respondents' experiences of the crematorium, as funeral and crematorium workers are usually trained to respond sensitively to bereaved people.

The following narrative demonstrates some of the more 'typical' every day social responses respondents encountered following their loss:

R: It wasn't as though it was painful to see them [mothers] with their babies but it was when they ran across the road and pretended they hadn't seen me. One woman in particular, she would always run away, literally run away. And one day I actually bumped into her in a shop doorway so she couldn't avoid me [laughs] and she tried to hide her baby behind her back, like literally. I had to say: 'who is this then?' with her hiding it behind her back. And she said: 'Oh this?' like oh where did this come from [laughs]. Oh God! .....I used to feel like I had tragedy literally tattooed on my forehead as I walked down the street and that every body knew even though they didn't. Sometimes I still feel like it, like I represented death to people all of a sudden and they couldn't handle it. Sometimes you get a good reaction, sometimes you get stunned silence and sometimes you get rubbish reactions................
Wynnie, mother of baby boy Bryn (stillborn at forty weeks).

In the previous account, it could be argued that the avoidant mother felt uncomfortable with the parent whose baby had died for several reasons. For example feeling guilty that her baby lived whilst another died. The response also suggests that infant death is relatively unfamiliar in people's own social network. When confronted with the real possibility that it has happened to someone they know it is too uncomfortable to bear. Indeed while society is exposed to these sad facts, discussion about how to cope if a loved one died is perceived as morbid and as though one is tempting fate (Walter, 1991). This notion concurs with parents accounts:

R: It is a parent's worst fear. So to know that it can actually happen and it's happened to the person standing in front of you is very scary. Also because when a baby dies it's not the person that everybody has known, it can be very hard for people to understand that you've lost a real person if they haven't seen them. I've noticed people with my photograph of Bryn [baby who died]. If I show it, it suddenly makes a much bigger impact because it's like Oh yeah he's real, he was a real baby...........................
Wynnie, mother of baby boy Bryn (stillborn at forty weeks).

This account reinforces the idea that the public expression of grief is at best considered morbid being too painful to witness.

232

This account also suggests that due to the increasing longevity of family members, people, in particular those who occupy higher socio economic groups, have high expectations of living a long life. Of note is the tendency of society to make heroes of people who are unable to prevent their own *untimely* death yet who try to raise public awareness about the fact that people die. For example the recent death of a young celebrity mother following a terminal illness prompted an increase in cervical cancer screening among young women in the UK.

Where previously people may have feared mortality, this has been replaced by anxieties surrounding the causes of death and preventative strategies. This shift in anxieties argues Bauman (1992), represents the widely held belief in the west that since death has a specific cause it is somehow avoidable. Moreover hospitals and undertakers reinforce this sense of invulnerability by taking care of the dying and the dead away from the home and the community. Indeed, the majority of respondents in this study consulted with funeral firms to care for their baby's body prior to burial or cremation which suggests that social expectations governing ritual and mourning reflects a much more corporate endeavour.

The following account though an exception to this tendency demonstrates rituals which involve the whole family when a baby boy dies:

R: My Dad and my brothers made him a little coffin and my Mum lined it with some blue silk and wool, padded with sheep's wool and that was really lovely that they did that. My Dad picked him up [baby Bryn], because my dad wanted to put him into the coffin himself. The guy at the mortuary said he had never in all the years he'd been there, no one had ever come to collect their own child and that if it happened to his children he would have come himself. Why didn't more people do it? He couldn't understand why……..
Wynnie, mother of baby boy Bryn (stillborn at forty weeks).

The account demonstrates the extent to which the commonality of mortality is concealed. The man at the mortuary states that no one has *ever* collected their own child, instead leaving the body to be attended to by undertakers, a matter which left him clearly baffled.

This suggests that the majority of parents' were unaware or were not given the choice to collect their baby and bring them home. Indeed, Schott et al (2007: 194) argue that health professionals in some parts of the UK have been unwilling to release babies' bodies to parents, recommending instead that the baby is given to funeral directors'. They further argue (in their 2007 guidelines for health professionals in the event of a death of a baby) that there is no legal reason why parents should not be able to take their baby home prior to burial and that with appropriate advice (storing the body) they should be supported by staff if that is their wish.

In the following extract from the same narrative, the mother describes the importance of bringing her baby home since in the long term, it legitimized her grief to others who saw her baby and who shared in the ritual of mourning for her loss:

R: We brought him back here to this house, his body back here and he was here in this room. After ten days the whole house was full of flowers and cards that people sent just masses and masses. So we just put them all around his coffin, with candles. It meant that other people from the family, who hadn't come to the hospital, had the chance to come and see him as well…My best friend who was going to be a godmother was able to see him as well. In hindsight I just wish I'd invited loads more people to see him at that time, but I didn't know then, but I do wish I had. Because it was so good to show him to loads of people, because they all had a memory of him and from meeting other people. I know that's really hard, if nobody you know or your family saw your baby it just makes it more unreal for people…………

Wynnie, mother of baby boy Bryn (stillborn at forty weeks).

Of all the accounts, thus, far, Wynnie is the one parent who was able to create a memory of her baby in the minds of many friends and family by bringing her baby home for others to see him. Yet the uniqueness of this family's handling of events was that the baby was not treated as someone to be hidden. The baby was encouraged to be brought home by the baby's Nordic grandparents and extended family, each member of which shares a belief system which supports talking about death openly.

234

While this was not a situation experienced by the majority of respondents, it is useful to consider the public upsurge of emotion in response to the deaths of Princess Diana and the children who died in the Scottish Dunblane school massacre. These were deaths which clearly had an impact upon the public and suggest that society is able to handle death albeit from a distance. Furthermore, devastating events continue to occur and affect the public (recent 2009 Children in Need Appeal raised £65 million). Yet in an age where emphasis upon materialism, cosmetic perfection, fashion and affluence means that men and women of all ages are able to express a sense of youth and physical attractiveness, this only serves to postpone any reflection on personal mortality and of one's family members (Mellor and Shilling 1993; Bauman, 1992). Indeed, the following account demonstrates the difficulty others have in contemplating the death of a child:

R: I'm always very conscious to how other people will react to it because that is one of the hardest things, is other people's reactions... the people who shy away because they don't want to upset you or don't want to talk about it because it's uncomfortable for them and equally those who get very upset for you and start crying and you feel that you have to comfort them and it's just as hard................

Ruth. mother of baby girls Melody and Joy (born at twenty-seven weeks, lived for two hours).

In this account Ruth has to live with her loss in isolation whilst contemplating the emotional responses of some compared to the lack of others. Ruth's account was part of an interview in which she also spoke about the comfort she and her husband receive in regularly attending a religious service in the church where their daughters are buried. Of all the respondents, these parents are the only two people who have defined themselves as having any religious conviction.

Religious and Non-Religious Meaning

Where research has been undertaken to explore the relationship between religious explanations and meaning in the context of the death of a baby, this has largely been undertaken by people who hold strong religious beliefs. For example, Layne's (2003) American research respondents comprised of members of Compassionate Friends groups which were affiliated to religious institutions. This is in contrast with Cecil's (1994) study of Irish Catholic and Protestant women who held less fervent religious beliefs, and which may reflect an increasingly secularized society compared to its American neighbour. As with the subject of employment, respondents were not asked specifically about any religious beliefs they held unless the issue was brought up in the interview by men and women and explored further. Other than the two respondents identified, few men and women spoke about religion as a way of finding meaning to the death of their baby. Rather, respondents spoke about having a more personalised way of commemorating the baby's life even where they had engaged in a Christian service for their burial or cremation.

Several respondents spoke about memory boxes in which letters had been written by the mothers to their babies and of journals which tell the baby's story. Other respondents planted trees and bushes and carved out their own headstone to memorialise their baby. Words to mark the form of passing on headstones by respondents, for example, 'born and returned to the stars' and 'born asleep' (to signify a stillborn child) were also ways to humanise the more medical and socio-legal language assigned such deaths.

Respondent's creative endeavours could be explained as a means of having something to signify that the baby existed, other than the pre-planned nursery from which a toy or blanket could be held. Other men and women spoke about memorialising their baby by buying items such as cards and purchasing the services of an artist (through SANDS) who could draw a portrait of the baby who died from a photograph as a lasting memorial.

Items such as these were often referred to in interviews and shown which suggests that they help respondents to obtain some form of validation of their experiences. These largely secularised acts by respondents suggest that as with individual responses to loss, greater sensitivity needs to be afforded to the differences in the religious and non-religious needs of men and women following the death of a baby. This is a theme which is of particular relevance to respecting parents' needs when their baby dies in hospital.

Professional Discourse

Several respondents were unprepared for the possibility of a stillbirth or that their baby might die on the neonatal ward. Further, other than the pre-booked ultrasound scan few men and women had any experience of health professionals in hospital. Yet the role of midwives and doctors and their responses to patient's losses had a critical role in men's and women's experiences of the support they received. Several researchers attest to the fact that the care given to parents following perinatal loss can set the stage for the parents' entire grieving process both in the short and longer term (Schott, et al, 2007: 97; Leoni, 1997:361). In this study the responses of midwives and doctors served to either exacerbate a parent's distress or provide them with agency when they were treated with respect and sensitivity. The following account by a mother whose son was stillborn, demonstrates two very different approaches by consultants within the same maternity unit:

R: The Consultant Paediatrician and the consultant Obstetrician both came to see us , to talk to us, and um they were about as different as chalk and cheese really. One had a very different world view and um he was willing to say we just don't know what happened we can't understand it and we're so sorry, we just don't know basically. He also went further than that and said: 'Some people have a hundred years to live and some people have a fraction of a second who is to say which life is the more important.' An amazing thing to say at the time The other [second consultant], he just couldn't admit that we couldn't resuscitate him and he was saying: 'there'll be a reason and um we'll find out what it was. And if we hadn't have resuscitated him for that amount of time he would have had brain damage, it's probably for the best. It's probably better that he died.' Those were what his words were and um, I just withdrew inwardly and thought just Fuck off.....

...Well I think that it was I said. He just couldn't accept it, it was very defensive anyway, his kind of attitude. So I wasn't very impressed with him......
Wynnie, mother of baby boy Jack (stillborn at forty weeks).

This account demonstrates the varying responses which this respondent was exposed to and which in effect created two different modes of feeling and expression by the mother. The respondent is clearly touched by the sentiment offered by one consultant and repulsed by the insensitive comments of another. These responses occur within the same meeting with the mother yet differ markedly. There is the sad acceptance of the death by one consultant, yet a perceived failure by the other doctor. The latter response concurs with several authors' research on the responses of hospital staff to the death of a baby.

In Layne's (2003: 66-67) study on narratives of pregnancy loss, argues that the death of newborns represents the ultimate challenge to medical progress and to popularised notions of foetal and child development. Similarly, McHaffie and Fowlie (1996: 34) report similar findings. They argue that being unable to save a child's life represents a failure for many professionals who perceive their primary role as that of curing.

The findings suggest that the responses by some doctors does not imply a non-caring attitude, rather that medical training is centred upon therapeutic approaches to prolonging life.

Yet as Lovell states from her (1997:43) observations of health professionals and perinatal loss, midwives have a significant role in defining situations and shaping care.

This is demonstrated by the following account given by a mother of a baby girl Beth:

R: The thing that brought it all home for me was that a midwife came to see me and went through a tick list of what you do on discharge. I'd still got Beth there and she [midwife] said have you thought about contraception? And I said you are joking me, you are joking me, here I am holding Beth who's died and you're asking me about contraception, what planet are you on? She said: *'I've got to ask this'* and I said: 'no you don't.' Nobody showed any common sense, you know there are things on here that are just not appropriate to ask at the moment. It was just for something to say and it was easier and better for them to have a tick list that they could hide behind and not most of this isn't even relevant, I'm just going to use my common sense and obviously I've got to ask you about pain as those things are relevant....

Paula, mother of baby girl Beth (born at forty weeks, lived for seventeen hours).

The activity of the midwife in the previous account suggests that some staff feel obliged to tick and complete all boxes and columns on a detailed checklist. While this is a way of ensuring all the tasks to be carried out following loss are completed in British maternity and neonatal units, there is the danger that this is seen as a goal and an end in itself. Similarly Schott et al (2007:133) argue that such lists are unable to take into account the diversity of a parent's needs or when to discuss sensitive issues.

For Schott et al (2007: 133) checklists, especially those which pertain to the baby (seeing, holding, bathing, and dressing the baby) should function as a reminder to discuss these issues with men and women. Where this is lacking it is clearly distressing for some respondents. For example, in the following account this distresses concerns professional indifference to the loss:

R: I think the biggest thing for me was they didn't have a cot in all of the hospital they didn't have one and we had to put her in this rickety old pram......She ended up being put in a store cupboard in this pram; it was full of equipment, not a nice place to put our daughter. It was like well she's dead now so it doesn't really matter and that's how it felt. Everything just made our loss a hundred times worse because it was never acknowledged, the magnitude of the loss was never acknowledged, for us was never acknowledged by the people we were with.............

Paula, mother of baby girl Beth (born at forty weeks, lived for seventeen hours).

239

This account reflects that of other women in this thesis. Such insensitive and neglectful treatment of women makes a bad experience much worse. Moreover they support the need for ways to personify the baby in more humane ways.

Location of Care

Several researchers (Layne, 2005: 3; Lovell, 1997:39; Schott et al, 2007:101) have argued that the location of care can serve to either construct or deconstruct the identity of the mother and her child. For example, Schott et al, note that being able to labour in a single room for a deceased baby (died in the womb) is a critical factor in women receiving appropriate care. During interviews respondents discussed the location of their care in relation to bereavement suites (a room in which the parents can stay and dress, hold and have with their baby in privacy). While some respondents were afforded this facility, other respondents were not given the choice. The following accounts demonstrate varying experiences of the location of their care during and after labour:

R: In fact I ended up in a ward with a load of other Mums' with babies. I asked to be moved hence the put me up bed they put me in. That is one of my abiding memories is lying in a bed in a room with a load of other Mums' and their babies..... Which was not good................
Susie, mother of baby boy Billy (born at thirty-eight weeks, lived for nine hours).

R: I just wanted to smash her [midwife] face in just saying all the wrong things. It was just all clichés that were just completely wrong at the wrong time. It felt like I were in a play, playing a part that I didn't want to be in, and other people were just extras walking about and looking in. It was only then that they thought about putting us in a family room and they didn't have one. I can only describe it as .. it was like being ... it was like trying to put a round peg in a square ... we would never fit, we didn't fit into the rooms that they had and it was as if it was our fault... you've come in but actually we've got nowhere for you to go with your baby that has just died. It just made our grief and our loss so much harder because one, it was never acknowledged by the people involved and as a Mum that just crucifies you......

... There's no recognition as a life or how precious her life was to us...... It's a miracle of life but they seem to have no comprehension of that and they just become so blasé about life and death and it just felt all wrong .It was just.. nobody came to help us. I can only describe it as barbaric, there was no humanity, no integrity by the people involved and it crucified me. There was just never any depth to anything............
Paula, mother of baby girl Beth (born at forty weeks, lived for seventeen hours).

In this last account, several years have passed following the loss of her daughter. Yet it is evident to note the anger she feels when she refers to the health professional assigned to care for her as though the moment happened yesterday. Her experiences of the type of care she received and the location of that care served to exacerbate her distress. The mother's sense of rage and anguish are a response to the attitude of a professional which served to devalue her baby.

Similarly, the perceived sense of indifference by staff is demonstrated in the following narrative:

R: I was in the examining room and they just left me there. This one [nurse] I remember her coming in and she wanted....they were looking for a machine that they needed for another patient. There she was in our room so she was messing about with the wiring and everything and taking it out. She said to us, what have you had? I don't think she actually realised that in actual fact these are precious hours and we were just waiting for her [baby] to pass away...What makes me laugh is that I work with patients who are terminally ill and if a patient is admitted to a hospital ward they're given a cubicle, people stay away and they only go in if they need to. You wouldn't have somebody waltzing in Oh I'm borrowing this while you're about to die, you know, you respect that person dying and you allow the family to have some quality time with them on their death bed. When you have a baby it's like wayhay, you come in, have a look.....................
Sophia, mother of baby girl Elen (born at twenty-four weeks, lived for two hours).

This account demonstrates the importance of communication and of finding a way to notify members of staff that a baby is dying or has died and is with the parents in a particular room (e.g. colour coded symbol or note on the door). In the previous account, the nurse's presence in a room (usually reserved for examining patients) was innocent, yet there was evidently a lack of communication on the part of the maternity team.

241

While it could be assumed that midwives were busy, the lack of awareness of a dying baby and that of her mother who witnesses her dying is distressing.

This account reflects the indifference and relative lack of support afforded to the baby and her mother. Given the respondent's work as a nurse of the dying, she reflects on her situation with incredulity and disbelief. Sophia describes how her experience worsened due to the location of the examining room she birthed in since she was near a pay phone.

Sophia could over hear a phone conversation of the joyful sobs from a father relaying to the listener about the safe arrival of his baby boy, how much he weighed and the name he was going to call him. It is a memory which the respondent describes as one which sticks in her mind as though it happened yesterday. The relative lack of care for Sophia was encapsulated when she was discharged and sent home in under less than six hours following the birth and later death of her daughter.

These particular accounts were selected since they represented the negative aspects of other respondents care in hospital more generally. Together, the location of care, professional responses and institutional procedures in varying ways has negated these experiences. Similarly, Lovell's research (1997:39) found that health professionals played a key part in legitimizing or devaluing the meaning of the baby. These varying approaches it is argued extend to approaches to infant post mortem. The majority of respondents' children underwent this procedure to establish a cause of death, though for many, no explanation could be found.

These experiences prompted some women to attempt to sensitise the profession in one way by developing and conducting workshops with midwives.

At times, this provided a location in which these women told their stories and had the opportunity to suggest appropriate and more empathic responses which health professionals could employ with other bereaved parents. These types of activities were performed by several other women in this study alongside raising awareness of perinatal loss.

Baby Loss and Death Awareness

The death of a baby creates varying emotional reactions from others which suggests awareness about perinatal death is varying. The majority of respondents commented upon their own lack of awareness of baby loss prior to the death of their own child:

R: We didn't really know what to ask, we didn't have any information from SANDS or befrienders we didn't really know anyone apart from one couple and we didn't approach them. They had lost their baby six months before and my health visitor said they won't be ready to talk to you yet and we just accepted that. I was very naive and unquestioning. There was us in our little house and they were there in their little house and that's really sad......................

Lou, mother of baby girl Marie-Rose (stillborn, twenty-seven weeks).

Several respondents' previous awareness concerning perinatal loss was limited. For example, some men and women in interviews referred to their prior knowledge of infant mortality statistics and their sense of shock that their own child subsequently represented this mortal number. From this position, men and women gained a perspective and a body of knowledge which differed to that of a medical discourse. They tried to raise awareness and influence practice from membership of maternity liaison committees to engaging in political activities such as lobbying the Houses of Parliament (as part of SANDS activities in March 2009). Despite these activities, respondents continually assert in interviews that their grief remains delegitimized. There is no social script by which friends, family and colleagues can offer support generally.

243

Clearly, the issue of perinatal death needs a firmer public agenda. From respondents' accounts it also requires a critical evaluation of the way it is handled and managed by others. While not an insurmountable task the fact that deaths do occur needs to be more widely known and reported, in particular in pregnancy and birthing manuals, rather than '*ghettoised*' and confined to a page on the chapter on complications (Layne, 2003: 246). Indeed, the possible death of a baby needs to feature more widely in antenatal and childbirth classes and not glossed over for fear of upsetting pregnant women (Layne, 1990:71).

To this end, it is imperative that parents are forewarned of the possibility of a loss and informed about medical procedures and what they may expect. Indeed, respondents' accounts have highlighted this need. Yet with an over emphasis upon the promotion of new medical technologies to save and prolong life in science and the media people will continue to have unrealistic expectations. Consequently raising awareness around perinatal deaths is complex and needs to be handled sensitively and with a more measured account portrayed publicly which serves to demystify stillbirth and neonatal death.

Conclusion

In this fourth and final reading, some of the cultural and social structural contexts of parents' experiences following stillbirth and neonatal death have been explored. The dynamic by which parents renegotiate their sense of self is by transforming the representation of the baby to their inner and social worlds. As the reality that the child existed and died is shared and the parent's continuing bond with the child becomes a socially shared reality, the representation of the baby can be transformed into the parents' lives. This is not about an ending to grief and a severing of the bond with a dead baby, it is about integrating the child into the parent's life in a way which differed to when they were alive in the womb or on the neonatal ward. The ways in which the parent interacts with their child are varying but similar in purpose. The outcome is about finding a way to continue a bond with the baby and to show the child was a real baby, with real things.

The section on continuing bonds in this thesis represents a challenge to the prevailing theory in the bereavement literature which tends to support the view that the end point to grief is to sever ties with the deceased. This suggests that grief work needs to account for individual coping style, cultural diversity, and the differences inherent in the situational and death circumstances. Continuing a bond with the child is not only about renegotiating a relationship but making sense of others' responses to the death. Moreover, it is a way in which respondents reintegrate into the social world following the privacy of the family. These are ways to becoming accepted again while continuing a bond, which as one example demonstrated, was represented by the more physical task of parenting a grave.

Variations in response to the death of a baby and to parents' grief suggests that culturally and socially there are contradictory beliefs about how grief should be personally managed. It has been argued that current social and cultural beliefs and practice about death are inadequate in making sense of the loss of a child; in particular a baby that few people knew.

245

As a result parents may be treated with indifference and impatience and may feel the need to grieve alone and in isolation from others. As the section on employment suggests, respondents can be subjected to the insensitivity of colleagues at work as well as in wider society.

The lottery of empathic support is revealed in respondents' accounts about the location of their care and treatment by health professionals. Several respondents identified that where their care was supportive it was also lacking even within the same birthing unit. The expression of anger and despair by respondents in their accounts was notable as was the perceived indifference towards their care. This had implications in terms of personifying the baby and exacerbating the mother's distress both in the short and longer term. This seeming indifference extended to the way some babies bodies were treated after they had died.

An exploration of the social structures and cultural contexts within which men and women have discussed their experiences suggests that despite some profoundly negative experiences, parents are able to perceive what they view as social problems and issues (impatience by colleagues, insensitive sentiments and indifference from professionals). They offer their own possible solutions through political activity and targeting more sensitive professional practice and wider societal acknowledgement about the death of a baby.

The next chapter discusses key points from the four readings, and in view of existing literature about perinatal deaths and bereavement support, suggests recommendations for future research, and improvements in care.

CHAPTER 9. Conclusion

In this substantive research to understanding stillbirth and neonatal death, I have outlined a framework which incorporates the social in considerations of parents' experiences of grief and loss. In so doing, I have shown that these late modern experiences of bereavement are a reflection on the body, the self, and the destination to which life leads. The cultural power of these narratives is that their telling reveal voices of chaos nobody wants to hear since stillbirth and neonatal death lack the social endorsement that other deaths have. Yet these embodied experiences profoundly impact upon men and women's lives. While this impact is indeed similarly noted in the professional literature, it is unclear who this represents, the voices of professionals or the men and women affected.

What my analysis has demonstrated is the need for a personal voice to understanding experiences of grief and loss following the death of a baby. Such narratives are priceless since in calling to account men and women's perspectives of events, it has been possible to see narrations as a way into the complexity of voice and relationships.

These reveal embodied experiences of disillusionment for some, since it is not only what people say which seems harsh, but the realisation that fate is cruel. Indeed parents in this research think they have reached the limit of all possible suffering only to discover that suffering is limitless and that they could suffer more. Following dialogue with partners, family, colleagues and professionals they get to know about the social meaning of the death of a baby and learn that it is limiting. There is a general ambivalence which finds no reason for a body inhabited by the pain of loss and, thus, parents also learn that the resources for grieving are infinitely personal. In this respect, these men and women embody a parallel universe and one in which they live based on experience that few others can share.

Other ways of conducting research would not have enabled me to demonstrate the richness of these narratives. It is a novel approach which can be used in other studies to construct a comprehensive body of theory regarding men and women's bereavement experiences and which I have argued is missing from the literature concerning bereavement following stillbirth and neonatal death.

Indeed, the psychological understanding of this form of loss is problematic. For in providing overriding theories to explain bereavement, the varying categories of grief are conflated. Further, the pathology assigned to grieving men and women as defined by psychiatry is not based on research or clinical studies but upon cultural values from which the model emerged. I argued that the psychiatric sublimation of the uniqueness of the perinatal loss experience is therefore limiting since they do not fit with men and women's experiences in this research.

Further, I have argued that these dominant discourses do not fully explore other important mediating factors such as relationships with others and the presence of surviving siblings within the family. Yet these are critical to understanding varying parental responses to loss and to their sense of identity as a parent. Moreover, this sense of self is important in exploring ambivalent parental identity and social roles in this thesis.

It was from these social encounters that Giddens (1991) existential concerns to explain social responses to mortality were explored. Yet again this as with other theories was unable to assist in conceptualising the identity of the stillborn child or the baby who dies a neonatal death.

This research, therefore, provides a more adequate account of loss enabling men and women to describe how they experienced their grief following the death of their child and some of the ways they remain connected to their child in their daily life.

248

It can be seen that these continuing attachments represent a direct challenge to the stage theorists of grief who postulate the severance of ties to the deceased. In my study parents not only refuse to sever ties to their child they continue to parent, albeit in less overt ways.

In this reflexive approach to researching men and women's experiences of stillbirth and neonatal death, I have challenged the accepted traditional wisdom that somehow men and women 'get over' their loss and 'move on' without their child in their lives. In so doing, this research has expanded an understanding of bereavement beyond that of psychological and psychiatric theory and as one which can now be viewed as part of the ongoing parent's biography of their life.

Further, this research demonstrates men and women's desire to express their experience in the form of stories, journal entries, and poetry and commemorative passages on World Wide Web pages. Moreover, in the analysis chapters (5-8), I demonstrated that by reading and re-reading transcripts I was able to capture this discrete expressiveness by men and women which illuminated the strength of their loss. That this forms part of the data in this thesis shows what many other theoretical concerns have been unable to, which is to suggest that story telling represents an oral discourse.

While this approach to research was labour intensive, the process of reading and re-reading transcripts foregrounded a different aspect of the narrative and enabled reflexivity. With the use of my 'self' in research, I ensured that my role in the construction of data did not disappear which is an otherwise oft cited criticism of qualitative research.

By placing respondents and my 'self' at the centre of this research process, I have shown how reflexive sociology is a theoretical and a practical possibility. I have demonstrated that auto/biography in research is more than a recollection of events but a revaluation of the researcher's 'self' in the research process and how this has impacted upon the product.

249

This has been arrived at through a heuristic process leading to deeper connections with the subject matter. Indeed, by including my 'self' in this research, I have gained important insight into the relationship between the respondent and researcher and the challenges represented by 'insider' and 'outsider' identities. In so doing, it is possible to argue that this way of researching is not only insightful but also essential in considering the influence of the researcher to the research process and product. I made a case that critical self awareness provided an essential way of assessing the achievements and shortcomings of the voice relational approach to research.

While previous researchers have mentioned including their selves in research, I have argued that this has been under explored. Indeed, while Mauthner and Doucet (1998) and Brown and Gilligan (1992) before them have provided a way to understand experience, the reading and re-reading of data from interviews felt limiting since I wanted to capture what is not said in interviews.

This particular approach to my analyses demonstrated that while there were respondents who were reflexive, there were others who struggled with something to say. I showed that by listening to and capturing silences, I was able to expose the impact of such loss. For where there was a struggle to find words to accompany experience they said as much in their silence for these stories can be hard to tell.

This is often overlooked in the psychological understanding of grief. Similarly, other more sociological orientations permit a limited understanding about the way these stories are told, focusing instead upon the visceral tendencies of embodied emotions.

By including other forms of expression (poetry, narrative passages from journals, photographs) within interviews, the analysis revealed varying expressive preferences. For example, I presented a poem by a mother whose hospital experience was overwhelmingly negative (see p.186). This poetry needed few words to capture an experience; it revealed quite graphically the feelings, the experience, sense of powerlessness, stigma and shame the mother endured.

Other tangible representations of experience have been described within this thesis in the form of art and photographs (shown as part of interviews) and which the reader can interact with beyond that reached by the written word alone. Thus, the product of the research, whether a poem, a narrative or photograph was not a statement but a way of inviting respondents to consider what they think their experience is about and the medium by which this can be shared. These creative elements to the research have given the data a dimension that conveys the intellectual, bodily and emotional qualities of the experiences being studied.

In this approach to researching grief and loss I have been able to expose the variability of subjective experiences concerning perinatal death and its impact upon parents. While I could not know prior to research all the possible forms of experiences that respondents had, it meant I could include them. For example, the feticide narrative (p.152) represented a posteriori conceptualisation that was developed when the reading of the interviews was over. It was a narrative I had not expected since it represented one sub-narrative in a story about feticide, the central plot of which was the death of a child. Yet, how this came about as with others in this thesis, varied.

It is this consideration of loss which is missing in the multidisciplinary and professional literature concerning bereavement. Specifically I have been able to rethink the significance of these differences between respondent's accounts and between stillbirth and neonatal death.

251

Previous accounts of loss seemed to gloss over these differences and assume that these inequalities owe as much to a professional hierarchy of grief. I have now demonstrated how those very differences must be seen as part of the macro level of the institution bearing down on the micro level of emotion.

A particular dearth in the perinatal loss and health professional literature relates to the impact on men and on other family members in that they are barely mentioned at all. Yet for these individuals, it can be seen that the death represents a tragic disruption to their biography as well as that of the mother's.

The findings of this study serve to inform existing sociological theories. The differential experiences of men and women as mediated by social constructions of motherhood and fatherhood add to the research on gender that recognises the plurality of masculine and feminine identities in men and women. What I expose here is that occupation of this ambiguous role is consequential for identification as a bereaved parent, since they cannot be bereaved if they have not been a parent. In the eyes of others around them, they are not a parent, never having fulfilled that role more socially and it is this which makes it difficult (other than the physical representation of grief) for others to consider them bereaved. This view of self provides a way of understanding what men and women experience as lost when their child dies. I have demonstrated that it is these self stories which address respondent's situation since they call people to the identities they encapsulate. To this end the narrator (the parent in the interview) is telling the story while waiting to discover what other selves were operating unseen in the story that is their own.

Each self story in this thesis represents a form of narrative wreckage with each in its own way attempting to reclaim an original experience. Yet while the resources for reclaiming these stories are a product of the late modern age as presented on the World Wide Web and in support groups, they also contribute to their wreckage and to silencing grieving voices (i.e. the temporary cessation of the SANDS chat room, p.110) Though this exposes the inherent dangers of cyber communication it is nevertheless, original to this research. The counselling and professional literature does not generally expose the impact of these more negative electronic interactions and encounters.

It is possible to argue that these means of web based support are an imperfect solution. Much like support groups', discussion concerning stillbirth and neonatal death occurs after the event. This has far reaching implications for those men and women who learn that such things happen, only when it happens to them. Despite SANDS and bereaved parents' efforts in raising awareness, particularly in relation to stillbirth, there is still much less written about in terms of the impact of neonatal death, and as a consequence it contributes to the isolation that attends these events. Yet, as parents accounts in this thesis have shown the impact of such deaths needs to be viewed in a much more complex light and in relation to the cultural and social milieu to which men and women belong.

Indeed, what this thesis has shown is that we are now witnessing the emergence of a new paradigm for understanding death and social responses to the event. While religion and scientific discourse has sought to separate life from death, the new paradigm welcomes a closer relationship to finding meaning to mortality. This follows from an increasingly socially and culturally diverse Western society in which new beliefs are being traded for dissatisfaction with the old. Though some of these beliefs and practices such as continuing bonds have been around for some time, they have been marginalised by the dominant frameworks of modernity and, thus, represented abnormal behaviour.

To this end, both professionals and researchers need to give up the idea of trying to understand grieving men and women in the context of neat stages to be observed through. Moreover, it is an understanding which needs to be incorporated into the medical and nursing school curriculum in addition to ongoing professional development. That this needs to be applied consistently and nationally is evident in the lottery of care respondents have received and even with the same hospital.

I suggest that just as there are nursing consultants for specific areas of expertise such as dementia in the UK health system, so there is a scope as well as a need for bereavement midwives to train and receive support to deliver sensitive, compassionate care to grieving men and women.

Despite this, researchers need to continue to deconstruct the notion of stillbirth and neonatal death from its current form so that the varying needs of men and women can be identified and provision provided which reflects their gendered, ethnic, socio-economic, and situational needs. Indeed, since this research has shown that men are much less written about than women, future research agendas need to redress this balance for men's experiences to be accounted for. These experiences extend to other family members but research concerning the effects on these individuals is limited. Moreover, this research has shown that the impact of stillbirth and neonatal death is long lasting and again the long term effects need to be further explored.

In conclusion, this thesis demonstrates the extent to which both men and women's experience of stillbirth and neonatal death remains sequestered theoretically and practically. It is a body of research which is innovative in its understanding of men and women's embodied lived experiences and has practical implications for health care provision and the theoretical application of working with the bereaved. By its design, it contributes and lends weight to further development of a critical sociological death debate that engages with research and theory.

Further, it contributes to a multidisciplinary body of research and has implications for understanding experiences of perinatal loss, policy application and future research developments.

I finally end this thesis as I have started – on a reflexive note. Throughout this research, the voices of bereaved men and women have been heard and the impact of their loss profoundly expressed and presented.

In writing this thesis, I have found a location for my own voice as a researcher and as a woman who has witnessed the death of my child. That my daughter would be ten this year and playing with her sister and brother means that she continues to exist for in so many ways and in so doing, continues to be an evolving part of my family's biography and she will remain so until the last.

Bibliography

Aho, A.L., Tarkka, M.T., Kurki, P.A., Kaunoen, M. (2009) Father's experience of social support after the death of a child. *American Journal of Men's Health,* 3 (2), 93-103.

Archer, J. (1999) *The Nature of Grief: The Evolution and Psychology of Reactions to Loss.* London: Routledge.

Ariès, P. (1974) *Western Attitudes toward Death from the middle Ages to the Present.* London: Allen Lane.

Ariès, P. (1981) *The Hour of Our Death.* London: Allen Lane.

Ariès, P. (1993) Death Denied. In D. Dickenson, and M. Johnson (Eds.) *Death Dying and Bereavement.* London: Sage.

Armentrout, D.C. (2005) *Holding a place: A grounded theory of parents bringing their infant forward in their daily lives following the removal of life support and subsequent infant death.* Unpublished Ph.D Thesis.The University of Texas Graduate School of Biomedical Sciences at Galveston, US.

Armstrong, D (1994) Bodies of knowledge/ knowledge of bodies. In C. Jones and R. Porter (Eds.) *Reassessing Foucault: Power, Medicine and the Body.* London: Routledge.

Arney, W.R. and Bergen, B.J. (1984) *Medicine and the Management of Living,* Chicago: University Chicago Press.

Ashurst, P. and Hall, Z. (1989) *Understanding Women in Distress.* London: Tavistock.

Attig, T. (1996) *How We Grieve: Re-learning the World.* New York: Oxford University Press.

Atkinson, P. (1995) *Medical Talk and Medical Work.* London: Sage.

Attig, T. (2001) Relearning the world: making and finding meanings. In R. Neimeyer. (Ed*.) Meaning reconstruction and the and the experience of loss.* American Psychological Association, Washington.

Baker, P.S., Yeols, W.C., and Clair, J.M.(1996) Emotional expression during medical encounters: social disease and the medical gaze. In V. James and J. Gabe (Eds.) *Health and the Sociology of Emotions.* Cambridge: Blackwell.

Bakhtin, M.M.(1984) *Rabelais and his World,* trans. H. Iswolsky. Bloomington: Indiana University Press.

Bauman, Z. (1992) *Mortality, Immortality and Other Life Strategies.* Cambridge: Polity Press.

Becker, E. (1973) *The Denial of Death. New York: Collier-Macmillan.*

Behar, R. (1996) *The Vulnerable Observer: Anthropology that Breaks Your Heart.* Boston: Beacon Press.

Benfield, D.G., Leib, S.A., and Vollman, J.H. (1978) Grief Response of Parents to Neonatal Death and Parent Participation in Deciding Care. *Pediatrics,* 62 (2), 171-177.

Bennett, G., and Bennett, K.M. (2000) The Presence of the Dead: an empirical study. *Mortality,* 5 (2), 139-157.

Berger, P. and Luckman, T. (1966) *The Social Construction of Reality.* Harmondsworth: Penguin.

Birdwhistell, R. (1970) *Kinesics and Context.* Philadelphia: University of Pennsylvania Press.

Blum, A., and McHugh, P. (1984) *Self reflection in the arts and sciences.* Atlantic Highlands, NJ: Humanities Press.

Bonanno, G.A., and Keltner, D. (1997) Facial expression of emotion and the course of conjugal bereavement. *Journal of Abnormal Pyshcology,* 106, 126– 137.

Boulton, D., and Hammerlsey, M. (1996) Analysis of Unstructured Data. In R. Sapsford and V. Jupp (Eds.) *Data Collection and Analysis.* London: Sage.

Bourne, S., Lewis, E. and Vallender, I. (1992) *Psychological aspects of stillbirth and neonatal death.* London: Tavistock Clinic.

Bowlby, J. (1980) *Attachment and Loss, Volume I. Loss, Sadness and Depression.* London: Pimlico and The Institute of Psychoanalysis.

Bowlby, J. (1998) *Attachment and Loss, Volume II. Separation and Anxiety.* London: Pimlico and The Institute of Psychoanalysis.

Braun, M.J. and Berg, D.H. (1994) Meaning reconstruction in the experience of parental bereavement.*Death Studies,* 18 (2), 328-46.

Brost, L. and Kenney, J. (1992) Pregnancy after perinatal loss: parental reactions and nursing interventions. *JOGN,* 21, 457- 463.

Brotheridge, C.M. and Lee, R.T. (2003) Development and validation of the emotional labor scale. *Journal of Occupational and Organisational Psychology,* 76, 7-19.

Brown, F.H. (1989) The Impact of Death and Serious Illness on the Family Life Cycle. In E. Carter and M. McGoldrick (Eds.) *A Framework for Family Therapy* (2nd edition). Boston. Allen and Bascon.

Brown, L.M., and Gilligan, C. (1992) *Meeting at the Crossroads: Women's Psychology and Girl's Development.* Massachusetts: Harvard University Press.

Bruner, J. (1990) *Acts of Meaning.* Cambridge, Mass: Harvard University Press.

Burck, C. (2005) Comparing qualitative research methodologies for systemic research: the use of grounded theory, discourse analysis and narrative analysis. *Journal of Family Therapy,* 27, 237-262.

Burr, J. (2009) Exploring reflective subjectivity through the construction of the 'ethical other' in interview transcripts. *Sociology,* 43 (2), 32-39.

Burr, V. (1995) *An Introduction to Social Constructionism.* London: Routledge.

Byrne, L. (2008) *Angels in my Hair.* London: Arrow Books

Caelli, K., Downie, J., and Letendre, A.(2002) Parents' Experience of Midwife Managed Care Following the Loss of a Baby in a Previous Pregnancy. *Journal of Advanced Nursing,* 39 (2), 127-136.

Cain. A.C., and Cain B.S. (1964) "On replacing a child." *Journal of the American Academy of Child Psychiatry* 3, 443-456.

Cecil, C. (1996) *The Anthropology of Pregnancy Loss.* Oxford: Berg.

Cecil, R. (1994) "I wouldn't have minded having a wee one running about": Miscarriage and the family. *Social Science and Medicine,* 38 (10), 1415-1422.

Chitty, D. (2009) *An Angel Set me Free.* London: Harper Element.

Coltrane, S. (2007)Fathering: Paradoxes, Contradictions and Dilemmas. In K.S., Kimmel, and M.A., Messner, (Eds.) *Men's Lives.* New York: Pearson.

Collins, R. (1990) Stratification, emotional energy, and the transient emotions. In T.J. Kemper (Ed.) *Research Agendas in the Sociology of Emotions.* New York: State University of New York Press.

Condon, J.T. (1986) Management of Established Pathological Grief Reaction After Stillbirth. *American Journal of Psychiatry,* 143, 987-992.

Cornwell, J. (1984) *Hard Earned Lives: Accounts of Health and Illness from East London*. London: Tavistock Publications.

Cote-Arsenault, D. (2003) Weaving babies lost in pregnancy into the fabric of family life. *Journal of Family Nursing*, 9 (23), 23-36.

Cotterill, P. (1992) Interviewing women: issues of friendship, vulnerability and power. *Women's Studies International Forum*, 15 (5/6), 593-606.

Craig, G., Corden, A., Thorton, P. (2002) Safety in Social Research. *Social Research Update*. Issue 29. http://www.soc.surrey.ac.uk/sru.SRU29. HTML.

Crossley, M. L. (2000) *Introducing Narrative Psychology: Self, Trauma and the Construction of Meaning*. Buckingham: Open University Press.

Darwin, C. (1872/1955) *The Expression of Emotions in Man and Animals*. New York: Philosophical Library.

Davies, J. (1996) Vile bodies and mass media chantries. In G. Howarth and C. Jupp. (Eds.) *Contemporary Issues in the Sociology of Death and Dying*. London; Macmillan.

Deal, J., Wampler, K., and Halverson, C. (1992) The importance of similarity in the marital relationship. *Family Process*, 31, 369-82.

De Beauvoir, S. (1972) *The Second Sex*. Harmondsworth: Penguin Books

De Frain, J.D., Martens, L., Stork. J., and Stork, W. (1990-1991) The Psychological Effects of Stillbirth on Surviving Family Members. *Omega*, 22, 81-108.

Dent, A. and Stewart, A. (2004) *Sudden Death in Childhood, Support for the Bereaved Family*. London: Butterworth, Heinemann.

Department of Health (2007) *Mortality Target Monitoring (Infant Mortality,*
Inequalities).http://www.dh.gov.uk/en/Publicationsandstatistics/DH06554. 13.11.09.

Dermott, E. (2008) *Intimate Fatherhood. A Sociological Analysis*. London: Routledge.

Descartes, R. (1637/1985) *The Philosophical Writings of Descartes*. Edited by J. Cottingham, R. Stoothoff, and D. Murdoch. Cambridge: Cambridge University Press.

De Swaan, A. (1990) *The Management of Normality: Critical Essays in Health and Welfare*. London: Routledge.

De Vries, B., Lana, R.D., and Falck, V.T. (1994) Parental Bereavement Over the Lifecourse: A Theoretical Intersection and Empirical Review. *Omega,* 29 (1), 47-69.

Dickens, C. (1848/1995) *Dombey and Son.* London: Penguin Books.

Dingwall, R. (1997) Accounts interviews and observations. In G. Miller and R. Dingwall (Eds.) *Context and Methods in Qualitative Research.* Thousand Oaks, California: Sage.

Don, A. (2005) *Fathers Feel too.* London: Bosun.

Douglas, M., and Calvez, M. (1990) The self as risk taker: a cultural theory of contagion in relation to AIDS. *Sociological Review*, 38, 445-64.

Dyregrov, A. (1990) Parental reactions to the loss of an infant child: a review. *Scandinavian Journal of Psychology,* 31 (4), 226-80.

Dyregrov, A., and Mathiessen, S.B. (1991) Parental grief following the death of an infant. A follow-up over one year. *Scandinavian Journal of Psychology*, 32 (3), 199-207.

Dyregrov, S. (2008) *Grief in Young Children. A Handbook for Adults.* London: Jessica Kingsley.

Eckman, P., Friesen, W.V., and Elsworth, P. (1972) *Emotion in the Human Face.* New York: Pergamon Press.

Ellis, C. and Berger, L. (2003) Their story/ my story/our story; Including the researcher's experience in interview research. In J.F. Gubrium and J.A. Holstein (Eds.) *Postmodern Interviewing.* Thousand Oaks, CA: Sage.

Elias, N. (1985) *The Loneliness of Dying.* Oxford: Blackwell.

Emery, J.L. (1990) Attitudes of parents and paediatricians to a baby's death. *Journal of the Royal Society of Medicine*, 83, 423-424.

Engel, G.I. (1961) 'Is grief a disease?' *Psychosomatic Medicine.* 23 (1) 18-22.

Enkin, M., Keirse, M.J., Neilson, J., Crowther, C., Hodnett, E., and Hofmeyr, J. (2000) *A guide to effective care in pregnancy and childbirth* Oxford University Press: Oxford.

ESRC (2007) *Research Ethics Framework, 2007.* Swindon: Economic and Social Research Council.

Etherington, K. (2004) *Becoming a Reflexive Researcher. Using ourselves in research.* London: Jessica Kingsley.

Etherington,K. (2006) Understanding drug misuse and changing identities; A life story approach. *Drugs, education, prevention and policy*, 13 (3) 233-245.

Feeley, N., and Gottlieb, L.N. (1988-1989) Parents' Coping and Communication Following their Infant's Death. *Omega*, 19, 51-67.

Fenwick, J., Jennings, B., Downie, J., Butt, J., and Okanaga, M. (2007) 'Providing perinatal loss care: Satisfying and dissatisfying aspects for midwives.' *Women and Birth*, 20 (4), 153-160.

Finkenbeiner, A. (1996) After the death of a child. Living with loss through the years. Baltimore: Johns Hopkins University press.

Fish, W.C. (1986) Differences of Grief Intensity in Bereaved Parents. In T.A. Rando (Ed.) *Parental Loss of a child*. Champaign, Illinois: Research Press.

Fontana, A. and Frey, J.H. (2000) The interview: From structured interviews to negotiated text. In N.K. Denzin and Y.S. Lincoln (Eds.) *Handbook of Qualitative Research* (2nd edition) Thousand Oaks, California: Sage.

Forrest, G.C., Standish, E., & Baum, J.D. (1982) Support after perinatal death: a study of support and counselling after perinatal bereavement. *British Medical Journal*, 285, 1475-9.

Foucault, M. (1975) *The Birth of the Clinic: An Archaeology of Medical Perception*. New York: Vintage Books.

Foucault, M. (1984) *Space, knowledge and power*. In P. Rainbow (Ed.) The Foucault Reader. New York: Pantheon

Frank, A. (1995) *The wounded storyteller: Body, illness and ethics.* Chicago: Chicago University Press.

Frankl, V.E. (2006) *Man's Search for Meaning*. Boston: Beacon Press.

Franklin, S. (1997) *Embodied Progress: A Cultural Account of Assisted Conception.* London: Routledge.

Freeman, M. (1993) *Rewriting the Self: History, Memory, Narrative.* London: Routledge.

Freeman, T. (2003) Loving Fathers or Deadbeat Dads: The Crisis of Fatherhood in Popular Culture. In S. Earle and G. Letherby (Eds.) *Gender, Identity and Reproduction.* Hampshire, London: Palgrave Macmillan.

Freund, P.(1990) The expressive body: a common ground for the sociology of emotions and health and illness. *Sociology of Health and Illness,* 12 (4), 452-77.

Freud, S. (1913/1957) Mourning and melancholia. In J. Strachey (Ed. and Trans) *The standard edition of the complete psychological works of Sigmund Freud.* Volume 14, 243-258. London: Hogarth Press.

Freud, S. (1917/1973) *Introductory lectures on psychoanalysis.* Hammondsworth: Penguin.

Frost, J. (2004) *Uncertain Age: Late Motherhood and Early Miscarriage.* Unpublished PhD Thesis. University of Bristol, Bristol, UK.

Gardner,J.M. (1999) Perinatal death: Uncovering the needs of midwives and nurses and exploring helpful interventions in the United States, England and Japan. *Journal of Transcultural Nursing,* 10 (2),120-130.

Garfinkel, H. (1967) *Studies in ethnomethodology.* Englewood Cliffs, New Jersey: Prentice Hall.

Gergen, K. (1994) *Toward Transformation in Social Knowledge.* (2nd edition). London: Sage.

Giddens, A, (1984) *The Constitution of Society: Outline of a Theory of Structuration.* Cambridge: Polity Press.

Giddens, A. (1991) *Modernity and Self- identity.* Cambridge: Polity Press.

Gilbert, M. (1985) *The Holocaust: A History of the Jews of Europe during the Second World War.* New York: Holt, Rineheart and Winston.

Giles, P.F.H. (1970) 'Reactions of Women to Perinatal Death'. *Australian and New Zealand Journal of Obstetrics and Gynecology,* 10, 207-210.

Glaser, B. and Strauss, A. (1967) *Time for Dying.* Chicago: Aldine.

Goffman, E. (1959) *The Presentation of Self in Everyday Life.* New York: Doubleday Anchor.

Goffman, E. (1967) *Interaction Ritual.* New York; Doubleday Anchor.

Good, B. (1994) *Medicine, Rationality, and Experience.* Cambridge: Cambridge University Press.

Gorer,G. (1955) The Pornography of Death. *Encounter.* October.

Gorer, G. (1965) *Death, Grief and Mourning in Contemporary Britain.* London: Cresset.

Greene, M. (2010) The dot.commemoration GENERATION. *The Mail on Sunday YOU supplement*, 21 March, 52-55.

Grout, L.A., and Romanoff, B.D. (2000) The myth of the replacement child: parents' stories and practices after perinatal death. *Death Studies*, 24, 93-113.

Gubrium, J.F. and Holstein, J.A. (1998) Narrative practices and coherence of personal stories. *Sociological Quarterly*, 39, 163-87.

Guillemin, J.H, and Holmstrom, L.L. (1986) *Mixed Blessings: Intensive Care for Newborns.* Oxford: Oxford University Press.

Handley, N. (1991) Death awareness and personal change, in C.Newnes (ed.) *Death, Dying and Society.* Hove and London: Lawrence Elbaum Associates

Hanusch, F. (2008) Graphic death in the news media; present or absent? *Mortality,* 13 (4), 301-317.

Harré, R. (1991) *Physical Being: A Theory for a Corporeal Psychology.* Oxford; Blackwell.

Harvey, S., Snowdon, C., and Elbourne, D. (2008) Effectiveness of bereavement interventions in neonatal intensive care: A review of the literature. *Seminars in Fetal and Neonatal Medicine,* 13 (5), 341-356.

Hedtke, L. (2002) Reconstructing the Language of Death and Grief. *Illness, Crisis and Loss,* 10 (4), 285-293.

Hindmarch, C. (1995) Secondary loss for siblings. *Child: Care Health and Development,* 21, 425-431.

Hochschild, A., R. (2003) *The Managed Heart. Commercialization of human feeling.* Los Angeles: University of California Press.

Hockey, J. (1997) Women in Grief: Cultural representation and social practice In D. Field, and J. Hockey (Eds.) *Death, Gender and Ethnicity*, pp 89 – 107. London: Routledge.

Hogan, N. and De Santis, L.(1992) Adolescent sibling bereavement: an ongoing attachment'. *Qualitative Health Research* 2 (2),159–77.

Holdsworth, C., and Morgan, D. (2007) 'Revisiting the generalised other; an exploration. *Sociology,* 41 (3), 401-17.

Howard, G.S. (1991) Culture tales: A narrative approach to thinking, cross– cultural psychology and psychotherapy. *American Psychologist,* 46 (3), 187-197.

263

Howarth, G. (2008) *Death and Dying. A Sociological Introduction.* Cambridge; Polity Press.

Howson, A. (2009) *The Body and Society. An Introduction.* Cambridge: Polity Press.

Hughes, P. and Riches,S. (2003) Psychological aspects of perinatal loss. *Current Opinion in Obstetrics and Gynecology,* 15 (2), 107-111.

Hunter, M. (1994) *Counselling in Obstetrics and Gynaecology.* London: British Psychological Society

Illich, I. (1977) *Limits to Medicine: Medical Nemesis. The Exploration of Health.* London: Penguin.
James, W. and Lange, C.G. (1922) *The Emotions.* Baltimore: Williams and Wilkins.

James, W. and Carl, L.G. (1922) *The Emotions.* Baltimore: Williams and Wilkins.

Jolly, H. (1975 a) How hospitals can help parents to bear the loss of a baby. *The Times,* 5 November.

Jolly, H. (1975b) The heartache in facing the facts of a stillborn baby. *The Times* 3 December.

Jolly, H. (1976) Family reactions to stillbirths. *Proceedings of the Royal Society of Medicine,* 69, 835-7.

Jones, E. (1957) *Life and Work of Sigmund Freud, Volume 3.* London: Hogarth Press.

Josselson, R., and Lieblich, A. (1993) *The Narrative Study Of Lives,* 1. Newbury Park: Sage

Josselson, R. (1996) On writing other people's lives: Self analytical reflections of a narrative researcher. In R. Josselson (Ed.) *Ethics and Process in the Narrative Study of Lives, Volume 4.* London: Sage.

Josselson, R., and Lieblich, A. (1999) *Making meaning of narratives.* Thousand Oaks, California: Sage.

Josselson, R. (2004) 'The Hermeneutics of Faith and the Hermeneutics of Suspicion'. *Narrative Inquiry,* 14 (1), 1-28.

Kavanaugh, K.(1997) Gender Differences Among Parents' Who Experience the Death of an Infant Weighing Less Than 500 grams at Birth. *Omega,* 35, 281-296.

Keaggy, B. (2002) *Losing You Too Soon. Finding Hope after Miscarriage or the Loss of a Baby.* Oregon: Harvest House.

Keeling, M., and Nielson, R. (2005)Indian women's experience of a narrative intervention using art and writing. *Contemporary Family Therapy,* 37 (3), 435-452.

Kellehear, A. (2007) *A Social History of Dying.* Cambridge: University Press

Kellner, K. and Lake, M. (1990) 'Grief counselling.' *In High Risk Pregnancy a Team Approach.* In R. Knuppel and J. Drukker (Eds.) W.B. Saunders: Philadelphia.

Kemper, T. (1990) Social relations and emotions: a structural approach. In T.J. Kemper (Ed.) *Research Agendas in the Sociology of Emotions.*New York; New York State University Press.

Kenyon, S. (2002) Responding when a baby dies. *Journal of Family Health Care*, 12 (3), 58.

Kersting A., Dorsch, M., Kreulich, C. Reutman, M., Ohrmann, P. and Baez, E. (2005) 'Trauma and grief 2-7 years after termination of pregnancy because of fetal anomalies a pilot study. *Journal of Psychosomatic Obstetrics and Gynecology* 26 (1), 9–14.

Kirkley-Best, E. (1981) *Grief in response to perinatal loss: An argument for the earliest maternal attachment.* University Microfilms: Ann Arbor, Michigan

Kirkley-Best, E., and Kellner, K.R. (1982) 'The forgotten grief: a review of the psychology of stillbirth'. *American Journal of Orthopsychiatry*, 52, 420-429.

Klass, D.(1996) The deceased child in the psychic and social worlds of bereaved parents during the resolution of grief in, D. Klass, P.R. Silverman and S.L. Nickman (Eds.) *Continuing Bonds* London: Taylor Francis.

Kohner, N., and Henley, A. (1997) *When a Baby Dies. The Experience of Late Miscarriage, Stillbirth and Neo Natal Death.* Stillbirth and Neonatal Death Society (SANDS) London: Pandora Press.

Kohner, N., and Thomas, J. (1995) *Grieving after the death of your baby.* The Child Bereavement Trust: Bucks.

Krueger, R., and Casey. M.A. (2000) *Focus Groups: A Practical Guide for Applied Research.* (3rd edition) London: Sage.

Kubler-Ross, E. (1997) *On Death and Dying.* New York: Touchstone Press.

Kvale, S. (1996) *Interviews: An Introduction to Qualitative Research Interviewing.* Thousand Oaks, CA: Sage

Lambeck, M. (1996) The Past Imperfect: Remembering as Moral Practice. In P. Antze and M. Lambeck (Eds.) *Tense Past; Cultural Essays in Trauma and Memory.* New York: Routledge.

Lang, A., Gottlieb, L.N., Amsel, R. (1996) Predictors of husbands' and wives' grief reactions following infant death: the role of marital intimacy. *Death Studies*, 20 (1), 33–57.

Langer, L.L. (1991) *Holocaust Testimonies: the ruins of memory.* London: Yale University Press

Lapadat, J.C., and Lindsay, A.C. (1999) 'Transcription in research and practice: From standardization of technique to interpretive positionings'. *Qualitative Inquiry,* 5 (1), 87-13.

Lasker, J.N. and Toedter, L.J. (1991) Acute Versus Chronic Grief: The Case of Pregnancy Loss. *American Journal of Orthopsychiatry*, 61 (4), 510–521.

Layne, L. (1990) Motherhood lost: cultural dimensions of miscarriage and stillbirth in America. *Women and Health.* 16 (3/4), 69–98.

Layne, L. (2003) *Motherhood lost. A feminist account of pregnancy loss in America.* London: Routledge.

Layne, L. (2005) 'A Women's Health Model for Pregnancy Loss: A Call for a New Standard of Care.' Paper given at 'Reproductive *Disruptions'* Conference, University of Michigan. May 19-22, 2005.

Lee, C., Slade, P., and Lygo, V. (1999) The influence of psychological debriefing on emotional adaptation in women following early miscarriage: A preliminary study. *British Journal of Medical Psychology,* 69, 47-58.

Lee, R. (1993) *Doing Research on Sensitive Topics.* London: Sage.

Leon, I.G. 'Reproductive Losses: A Clinical Practice Advisory on Cultural Influences.' Paper presented at the *Reproductive Disruptions: Childlessness, Adoption and Other Reproductive Complexities Conference.* Institute for Research in Women and Gender University of Michigan, MI, USA, May 19-22, 2005.

Leon, I.G. (1992) Perinatal loss. A critique of current hospital practises. *Clinical Pediatrics,* 31 (6), 366–74.

Leoni, L.C. (1997) The nurse's role: care of patients after pregnancy loss. In J.R. Woods, J.L.E Woods (Eds.) *Loss during Pregnancy or in the Newborn Period.* New Jersey: Janetti Publications.

Lerner, H., McClain, M.,Vance, J. (2002) SIDS Education in Nursing and Medical Schools in the United States. *Journal of Nursing Education,* 41(8), 353-355.

Letherby, G. (2003) *Feminist Research In Theory and Practice.*Maidenhead: Open University Press.

Littlefield, C.H. and Rushton, J.P. (1986) When a child dies: the socio-biology of bereavement. *Journal of Personality and Social Psychology*, 51, 797-802.

Littlewood, J., Cramer, D. Hoekstra, J. and Humphrey, G. (1991) Gender differences In parental coping following their child's death. *British Journal of Guidance and Counselling*, 19, 139-48.

Littlewood, J. (1992) *Aspects of Grief: Bereavement in Adult Life*, London: Tavistock/Routledge.

Lovell, A. (1983) Some Questions of Identity: Late Miscarriage, Stillbirth and Perinatal Loss. *Social Science and Medicine* 17, 755-761.

Lovell, A.(1997) Death at the beginning of life. In D. Field and J. Hockey and N.Small (Ed.) *Death, Gender and Ethnicity.* London: Routledge.

Lupton, D. (2000) Foucault and the Medicalisation critique. In A. Petersen and R. Bunton (Eds.) *Foucault, Health and Medicine*. London: Routledge.

Lupton, D. and Barclay, L. (1997) *Constructing Fatherhood: Discourses and Experiences.* London: Sage.

Lyon, M.L.,and Barbalet, J.M. (2003) Society's body; emotion and the "somatisation" of social theory. In T.J. Csordas. (Ed.) *Embodiment and Experience. The Existential Ground of Culture and Self.* Cambridge: Cambridge University Press.

Mahan, C.K., and Calica, J. (1997) Perinatal loss: considerations in social work practice. *Social Work Health Care*, 24 (3-4), 141–52.

Mair, M. (1989) *Beyond psychology and psychotherapy: A poetics of experience.* London: Routledge.

Malcarida, C. (1999) Complicated Mourning; The social economy of perinatal death. *Qualitative Health Research,* 9, 504-519.

Mandell, F., Wolfe, L. (1975) Sudden Infant Death Syndrome and Subsequent Pregnancy. *Pediatrics*, 56, 774-776.

267

Marris, P. (1991) The social construction of uncertainty. In C.M. Parkes, J. Stevenson-Hinde, and P. Marris (Eds.) *Attachment Across the Life Cycle.* London: Tavistock.

Marwitt, S.J., and Klass, D. (1996) Grief and the role of the inner representation of the deceased in, D. Klass, P.R. Silverman and S.L. Nickman (Eds.) *Continuing Bonds* London: Taylor Francis.

Mauthner, N., and Doucet, A. (1998) Reflections on a Voice Centred Relational Method. In J. Ribbens and R. Edwards. (Eds.) *Feminist Dilemmas in Qualitative Research: Public Knowledge and Private Lives.* London: Sage

McCarthy, and Doyle, E. (1989) Emotions are social things; an essay in the sociology of emotions. In D.D. Franks, E.McCarthy, E.Doyle (Eds.) *The Sociology of Emotions: Original Essays and Research Papers.* Greenwich, Conneticut/ London: JAI Press inc.

McCleod, J. (2008) *Introduction to Counselling, Third Edition.* Milton Keynes: The Open University Press.

McHaffie, H.E., and Fowlie, P. (1996) Life, Death and Decisions. *Modern Midwife,* 12, 34-35.

Mellor, P.A., and Schilling, C. (1993) Modernity, self identity and the sequestration of death, *Sociology,* 27 (3), 411-31.

Merlau-Ponty, M. (2001) *Phenomenology of Perception,* trans. C. Smith. London: Routledge.

Miller, T. (2005) *Making Sense of Motherhood* Cambridge: Cambridge University Press.

Minow, M., and Shanley,M.L. (1996) Relational rights and responsibilities: revisioning the family in liberal political theory and law. *Hypatia,* 11 (1), 4-29.

Mischler, E. (1991) Representing discourse: The rhetoric of transcription. *Journal of Narrative and Life History,* 1, 255-280

Moustakas, C. and Douglass, B.G. (1985) 'Heuristic inquiry: The internal search to know.' *The Journal of Humanistic Pyshcology,* 25, 3, 39-55.

Moustakas, C. (1990) *Heuristic Research Design, Methodology and Applications.* London: Sage.

Murphy, F.A., and Hunt, S.C. (1997) Early pregnancy loss: men have feelings too. *British Journal of Midwifery,* 5, 287-90.

Nadeau, J.W. (1998) *Families Making Sense of Death*. London: Sage.

Najman, J.M., Vance, J.C., Boyle, F., Embleton, G., Foster, B. & Thearle, J. (1993) The impact of child death on marital adjustment. *Social Science & Medicine*, 37 (8), 1005-10.

Neimeyer, R.A. (1999) Narrative Strategies in Grief Therapy. *Journal of Constructivist Psychology*, 12, 1-21.

Newell, R.(1993) Questionnaires. In N. Gilbert (Ed.) *Researching Social Life*. London: Sage.

Obholzer, A. (2005) The impact of setting an agency. *Journal of Health Organization and Management*,19(4), 297-303.

Ochberg R.L. (1994) Life stories and storied lives. In A. Libelich (Ed.) *Exploring Identity and Gender: The Narrative Study of lives'*. Thousand Oaks, California: Sage.

Office for National Statistics (2006) *Mortality Statistics:* Series DH3 No. 37. London: Office for National Statistics.

Okley, J. (1992) Anthropology and autobiography: participatory experience and embodied knowledge. In J.Okley and H. Callaway (Eds.) *Anthropology and Autobiography*. London: Routledge.

O' Leary, J. (2009) Never a simple journey. Pregnancy following perinatal loss. *Bereavement Care*, 28 (2), 12-24.

Parkes, C.M. (1986) *Bereavement: studies of grief in adult life*, London: Tavistock.

Parkes, C.M., Laungani, P. and Young, B. (1997) (Eds.) *Death, Dying and Bereavement Across Cultures*. London: Routledge..

Peppers, L.G., and Knapp, R.J. (1980) *Motherhood and Mourning: Perinatal death*. New York: Praeger.

Quiller-Couch, A. (Ed.) (1919) *The Oxford Book of English Verse*. Oxford; Clarendon Press.

Radley, A. (1989) Style discourse and constraint in adjustment to chronic illness. *Sociology of Health and Illness*, 11, 230-52.

Rando, T. (1991) Parental adjustment to the death of a child. In D. Papadatou and C. Papadatos (Eds.) *Children and Death*, New York: Hemisphere.

Raphael, B. (1983) *The Anatomy of Bereavement*. New York: Basic Books

Riches, G., and Dawson, P. (1997) Shoring up the walls of heartache: Parental responses to the death of a child. In D. Field and J. Hockey and N.Small (Ed.) *Death, Gender and Ethnicity.* London: Routledge

Riches, G. and Dawson., P. (2000) *An Intimate Loneliness. Supporting Bereaved Parents and Siblings. Buckingham: Open University Press.*

Rillstone, P. and Hutchinson, S.A. (2001) Managing the re-emergence of anguish: pregnancy after a loss due to anomalies. *Journal of Obstetric, Gynecologic, and Neonatal Nursing* 33(1), 64-70.

Roberts, H. (1981) *Doing Feminist Research.* London: Routledge and Kegan Paul.

Rodger, B. and Cowles, K. (1991) The Concept of Grief: an analysis of classical and contemporary thought. *Death Studies*, 15, 443-58.

Rogers, A. (1994) *Exiled Voices: Disassociation and Repression in Women's Narratives of Trauma.* Wellesley, Massachusetts: Stone Center Working Paper Series.

Rosaldo, R. (1989) *Culture and Truth: The Remaking of Social Analysis.* London: Routledge.

Rose, N.(1994) Medicine, history and the present. In C. Jones and R. Porter (Eds.) *Reassessing Foucault: Power, Medicine and the Body.* London: Routledge.

Rosenblatt, P. (2000) Parents' grief: narratives of loss and relationship. Philadelphia, PA: Brunner/Mazel.

Rosenthal, G. (2003) The healing effects of story telling: On the conditions of curative storytelling in the context of research and counselling. *Qualitative Inquiry*, 9 (6), 895-915.

Rubin, L.B. (2007) The Approach Avoidance Dance: Men, Women and Intimacy. In *Men's Lives* M.S. Kimmel and M.A. Messner (Eds.) 319-324. New York: Pearson

Rubin, S. (1984) Maternal attachment and child death; On adjustment, relationship and resolution. *Omega*, 15, 347-352.

Ruddick,S. (1989) *Maternal Thinking: Towards a Politics of Peace.* Boston, Massachusetts: Beacon.

Ruskin, D. (2002) *A Candle for Lisa*. Yorkshire: Pennine Pens

SANDS (2009) *Saving Babies Lives Report.* London: Stillbirth and Neonatal Death Society.

Sarbin, T.R. (1986) The narrative as a root metaphor for psychology. In T.R. Sarbin (Ed.) *Narrative Psychology: The Storied Nature of Human Conduct*. New York: Praeger.

Schatz, B.D. (1986) Grief of fathers. In T.A. Rando (Ed.) *Parental Loss of a Child*. Champaign, Illinois: Research Press.

Scherer, K.R. (1984) On the nature and function of emotion. In K.R. Scherer and P. Eckman (Eds.) *Approaches to Emotion*. Hillsdale, New Jersey: Lawrence Erlbaum and Associates.

Schiff, H. (1977) *The Bereaved Parent*. Crown: New York

Schildrick, M. (1996) Posthumanism and the Monstrous Body. *Body and Society*, 2 (1), 1-16.

Schilling, C. (1997) *The Body and Social Theory*. London: Sage.

Schott, J., Henley, A., and Khoner, N. (2007) *Pregnancy loss and the death of a baby. Guidelines for professionals.* London: Bosun Press.

Schwab, R. (1992) Effects of a child's death in the marital relationship: a preliminary study. *Death Studies*, 16, 141-54.

Seale, C. (1998) *Constructing Death. The sociology of dying and bereavement.* Cambridge: Cambridge University Press.

Seale, C. (2003) *Sudden death processing: an ethnographic study of emergency care*. Unpublished PhD thesis, Durham, University, UK.

Segal, N.L., Wilson, S.M., Bouchard, T.J. and Gitlin, D.G. (1995) Comparative grief experiences of bereaved twins and other bereaved relatives. *Personality and Individual Differences*, 18 (4), 511-24.

Seidler, V. (2004) Transforming masculinities: Bodies, power and emotional lives. In A. Boran and B. Murphy (Eds.) *Gender in Flux*. Chester; Chester Academic Press.

Shakespeare, W. (1598/2005) *Much Ado About Nothing*. London: Penguin Books.

Shakespeare, W. (1606/2005) *Macbeth*. London: Penguin Books.

Silverman, D. (1993) *Interpreting qualitative data. Methods for analyzing talk, text and interaction.* London: Sage.

Silverman, P.R., and Klass, D. (1996) Introduction: What's the Problem. In D. Klass, P. Silverman, and S.L. Nickman (Eds.) *Continuing Bonds*. London: Taylor and Francis.

271

Silverman, P.R. (2000) *Never Too Young to Know. Death in Children's Lives*. Oxford: Oxford University Press.

Simmonds, W. and Rothman, B. K.(1992) *Centuries of Solace: Expressions of Maternal Grief in Popular Literature*. Philadelphia: Temple University Press.

Simms, M. (1971) The Abortion Act after three years. *Political Quarterly*, 42 (3), 269-287.

Simms, (1981) Abortion after the myth of the Golden Age. In B. Hutter and G. Williams (Eds.) *Controlling Women: The Normal and the Deviant*. London: Croom Helm.

Smith, A. and Kleinman, S. (1989) Managing emotions in medical school; students contacts with the living and the dead'. *Social Psychology Quarterly*, 55, 56-69.

Snyder, C.R. (1997) Unique invulnerability: a classroom demonstration in estimating personal mortality. *Teaching of Psychology*, 24, 3,197-9.

Sorensen, R. and Iedema,R. (2009) Emotional labour: clinician's attitudes to death and dying. Journal of Health Organization and Management, 23 (1), 5-22.

Stacey, J. (1997) *Teratologies: A Cultural Study of Cancer*. London: Routledge.

Stacey, J. (1991) Can there be a feminist ethnography? In S.B. Gluck and D. Patai (Eds.) *Women's Words, Women's Words: The Deminist Practice of Oral History*. New York: Routledge.

Statham, H. (2002) Prenatal diagnosis of fetal abnormality: the decision to terminate the pregnancy and the psychological consequences. *Fetal and Maternal Medicine Review*, 13, 213–247.

Stroebe, M. (1992) Coping with Bereavement: a review of the grief work hypothesis. *Omega*, 26 (1), 19-42.

Stroebe, W., Stroebe, M., Abakoumin, G., and Schut, H. (1996) 'The role of loneliness and social support in adjustment to loss: a test of attachment versus stress theory'. *Journal of Personality and Social Psychology*, 70 (6), 241-9.

Talbot, K. (1997) Mothers now childless: structures of the life-world. *Omega*, 36 (1), 45-62.

Tappan, M. (1997) Analyzing stories of moral experience: Narrative, voice, and the dialogical self. *Journal of Narrative and Life History*, 7, 379-386.

Thompson, J. (1984) Communicating with patients. In R. Fitzpatrick, J. Hinton, S. Newman, G. Scambler, and J.Thompson (Eds.)*The experience of illness.* London: Tavistock.

Thompson, N. (1997) Masculinity and Loss. In D. Field and J. Hockey (Eds.) *Death, Gender and Ethnicity.* London: Routledge

Toller, P.W. *(2005)* Negotiation of dialectical contradictions by parents who have experienced the death of a child. *Journal of Communication Studies,* 33, 46-66.

Tolman, D. (1992) 'Voicing the body: a psychological study of adolescent girls' sexual desire'. Unpublished PhD dissertation. Harvard University, Cambridge, Massachusttes.

Tronto, J. (1995) Care as a basis for radical political judgements. *Hypatia,* 10 (2),141-9.

Turner, K. (1982) Contemporary Feminist Rituals. In C. Spretnak. (Ed.) *The Politics of Women's Spirituality.* Garden City, New York: Anchor Books.

Turner, B.S. (1992) *Regulating Bodies: Essays in Medical Sociology.* London; Routledge.

Turner, J.H. (2007) *Human Emotions. A sociological theory.* London: Routledge.

Turner, J.H., and Stets, J.E. (2009) *The Sociology of Emotions*. Cambridge: Cambridge University Press.

Turton, P., Hughes, P., Evans, C.D., & Fainman, D. (2001) Incidence, correlates and predictors of post-traumatic stress disorder in the pregnancy after stillbirth. *British Journal of Psychiatry*, 178, 556-60.

Vance, J.C., Boyle, F.M., Najman, J.M., and Thearle, M.J. (1995) 'Gender Differences in Parental Psychological Distress Following Perinatal Death or Sudden Infant Death Syndrome'. *British Journal of Psychiatry*, 167, 6, 806-11.

Volosinov, V.N.(1986) *Marxism and the Philosophy of Language.* London: Harvard University Press.

Wallerstedt, C. and Higgins, P. (1996) Facilitating perinatal grieving between the mother and the father. *JOGNN,* 25, 389-394.

Wallerstedt, C., Lilley, M. and Baldwin, K.(2003) Interconceptional counselling after perinatal and infant loss. *Journal of Obstetric, Gynecologic and Neonatal Nursing,* 32 (4), 533-542.

Walter, T. (1991) Modern death: taboo or not taboo? *Sociology,* 25 (2), 293-310.

Walter, T. (1994) *The Revival of Death.* London: Routledge.

Walter, T.(1996) 'A New Model of Grief'. *Mortality,* 1 (1), 7-25.

Walter, T. (1999) *On Bereavement. The Culture of Grief.* Buckingham: Open University Press.

Way, N. (1994) In their own words: listening to inner-city adolescents speak their worlds. Unpublished PhD dissertation. Harvard University, Cambridge, Massachusetts.

Wengraf, T. (2001) *Qualitative Research Interviewing: Biographic Narrative and Semi - Structured Method.* London: Sage.

Williams, S.J., and Bendelow, G. (1996) Emotions, health and illness: 'the missing' link. In V. James and J. Gabe (Eds.) *The Sociology of Emotions.* Cambridge, Massachusetts: Blackwell.

Woodward, K. (2003) Representations of Motherhood. In S. Earle and G. Letherby (Eds.) *Gender, Identity and Reproduction.* Hampshire: Palgrave Macmillan.

Worden, J, W. (1991) *Grief Counselling and Grief Therapy (second edition).* London: Routledge.

Worden, J, W. (2003) *Grief Counselling and Grief Therapy (third edition). A Handbook for the Mental Health Practitioner.* New York: Brunner – Routledge.

Wortman, C., and Silver, R. (1989) The myths of coping with loss. *Journal of Consulting and Clinical Psychology,* 57 (3), 349-57.

Worth, N.J. (1997) Becoming a Father to a Stillborn Child. *Clinical Nursing Research,* 6, (1), 71-89.

Wright, R. (1994) *The Moral Animal: Evolutionary Psychology and Everyday Life.* New York: Pantheon.

Younnis, J. (1980) *Parents and peers in social development: A Sullivan-Piaget perspective.* Chicago: University of Chicago Press.

Zeanah, C.H. (1989) 'Adaptation following perinatal loss: a critical review'. *Journal of American Academic Child and Adolescent Psychiatry*, 28 (4), 467-80.

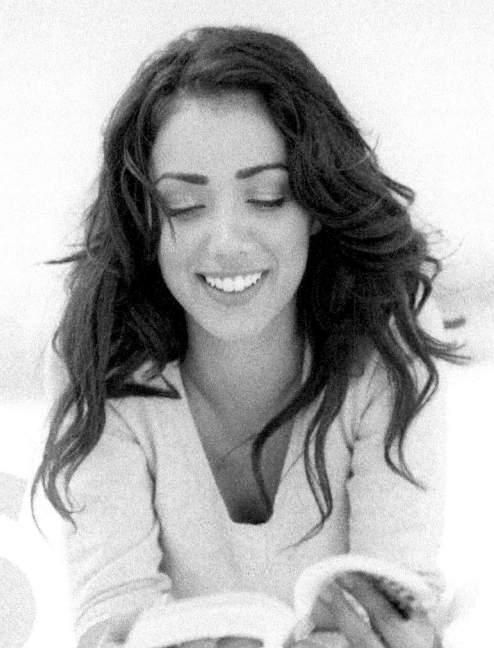
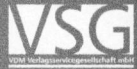

Lightning Source UK Ltd.
Milton Keynes UK
UKHW012352210421
382415UK00001B/14